THE MINI ADHD COACH

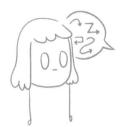

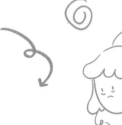
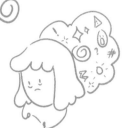
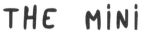
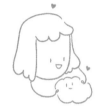

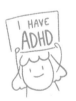
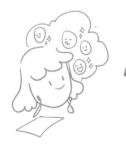

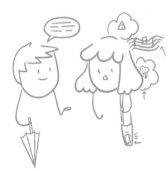

THE MINI
ADHD
COACH

Tools and Support
to Make Life Easier
A VISUAL GUIDE

Alice Gendron

CHRONICLE PRISM

First published in the United States of America in 2023 by Chronicle Books LLC.
Originally published in Great Britain in 2023 by Vermilion.

Library of Congress Cataloging-in-Publication Data available.

ISBN 978-1-7972-2733-7

Manufactured in China.

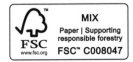

MIX
Paper | Supporting
responsible forestry
FSC™ C008047
FSC
www.fsc.org

This book contains advice and information relating to health and interpersonal
well-being. It is not intended to replace medical or psychotherapeutic advice and
should be used to supplement rather than replace any needed care by your doctor
or mental health professional. While all efforts have been made to ensure accuracy
of the information contained in this book as of date of publication, the publisher
and the author are not responsible for any adverse effects or consequences that
may occur as a result of applying the methods suggested in this book.

10 9 8 7 6 5 4 3 2 1

Chronicle books and gifts are available at special quantity discounts to corporations,
professional associations, literacy programs, and other organizations. For
details and discount information, please contact our premiums department
at corporatesales@chroniclebooks.com or at 1-800-759-0190.

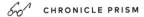

CHRONICLE PRISM

Chronicle Prism is an imprint of Chronicle Books LLC
680 Second Street, San Francisco, California 94107

www.chronicleprism.com

What's wrong with me?

For many years I asked myself these questions:

- Why can't I stay consistent when I start a new hobby?
- Why can't I control myself and avoid interrupting people when they talk?
- Why can't I stay on top of my work or my homework?
- Why can't I pay my bills on time?
- Why can't I remember to go to my dentist appointment?
- Why can't I keep a plant alive?

These questions started to pop into my head when I was a kid, and they kept getting louder and louder. At the start of my twenties, the questions were perturbing. In my late twenties, they started to feel very upsetting. In the end, the one question that summarized them all was: "What's wrong with me?"

Now I know. The answer is: nothing. Nothing is wrong with me. My struggles and my behavior are perfectly normal… for someone with ADHD.

Getting diagnosed at 29 and being able to share my challenges with my online community helped me realize this. Among people with ADHD, my "quirks" are the norm, and my weirdest anecdotes are perfectly ordinary.

Looking back, my ADHD was obvious all my life. I was a creative child who got in trouble for talking too much and acting impulsively. I was a dreamy teenager, able to focus for hours on my artwork, but not able to fully pay

MANY TIMES THROUGHOUT MY LIFE

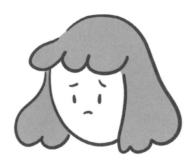

I WONDERED IF SOMETHING WAS WRONG WITH ME

attention to what my teacher was saying in class. I was a confused young adult, jumping from one career to another, and accumulating late fees for every bill. For months I fought the idea of getting assessed, before I finally found the courage to ask for an assessment appointment. I was terrified of being dismissed. I was convinced I was making it up. But I needed answers so badly that I did it anyway.

When the psychiatrist who assessed me casually remarked, "It's quite obvious that you have ADHD," I felt a weight lift from my shoulders. I knew that from that moment, I would be able to stop asking myself, "What's wrong with me?" every day. I had an answer. I had something to research and understand. And most importantly, I wasn't alone anymore.

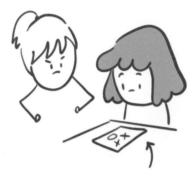

WHEN I WAS MAKING TOO MANY MISTAKES AT SCHOOL...

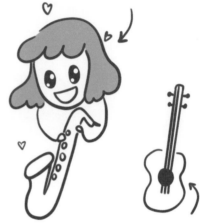

...BUT NOT SO MUCH ABOUT PERSEVERING

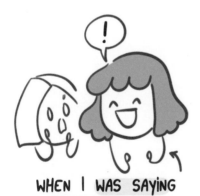

WHEN I WAS SAYING THINGS IMPULSIVELY...

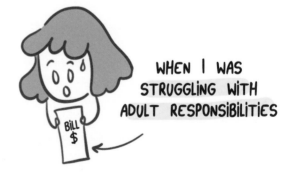

WHEN I WAS STRUGGLING WITH ADULT RESPONSIBILITIES

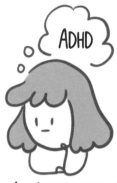

THEN I DISCOVERED ADHD AND I STARTED TO WONDER IF I COULD HAVE IT...

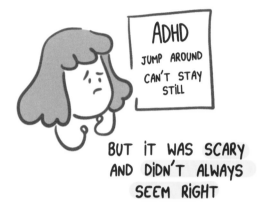

BUT IT WAS SCARY AND DIDN'T ALWAYS SEEM RIGHT

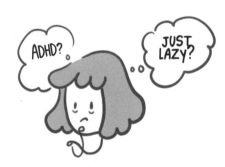

I LIVED WITH DOUBTS FOR MONTHS BEFORE I DECIDED TO SEE A PROFESSIONAL...

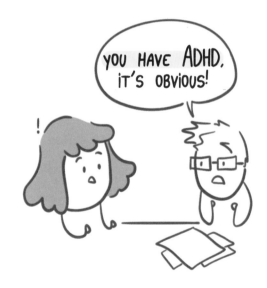

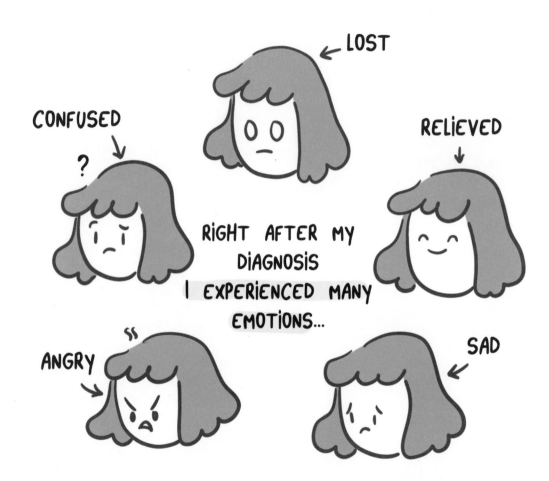

How to use this book

When I started posting doodles about ADHD on Instagram in 2020, I just wanted to share my experience in order to start conversations. Almost instantly, many people told me how relatable my drawings felt to them. They said my doodles helped them feel less alone with their quirks and struggles.

I want this book to bring you the same feeling. I would like you to understand that what is normal for others may not be normal for you, and vice versa. Whether you have already been diagnosed, or are just starting your journey, I hope that reading this book will help you realize that nothing is wrong with you. Your feelings are valid, and your struggles are real. You just need to understand yourself better.

If you are reading this book because you know someone with ADHD and you want to understand them better:

Congrats! You are a good friend. Having people around us willing to listen and to understand what we experience is vital. This book will help you understand what it's like to live with ADHD, and what can help us manage our symptoms.

This is a book about ADHD, made by someone with ADHD. So feel free to open and read it from a random page, start it from the end, zone out and re-read the same paragraph ten times in a row, or avoid the pages that you don't want to read.

PART 1

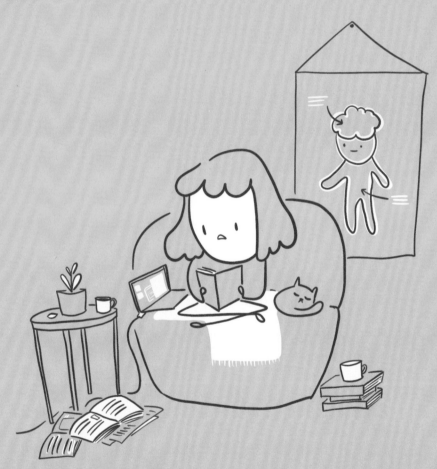

ADHD is a very misunderstood condition. There are many misconceptions surrounding ADHD, and it deserves to be better understood, especially by those who live with it. Understanding how our brains work and what challenges these differences typically bring is the key to finally feeling at peace. When we know why we act the way we do, it's much easier to find a solution; when we know we're not alone in acting this way, it's much easier to develop kindness towards ourselves.

ADHD 101

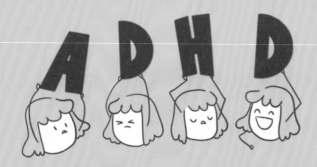

WHAT IS ADHD?

CHAPTER 1

What is ADHD?

Being diagnosed with ADHD doesn't mean that you instantly know what ADHD is. I receive messages every day from people telling me they were diagnosed in childhood, but didn't realize the impact ADHD had on their daily lives. When I was diagnosed aged 29, I felt the same. I was told I had ADHD, but no one ever explained what this meant. So let's take a look at what ADHD really is!

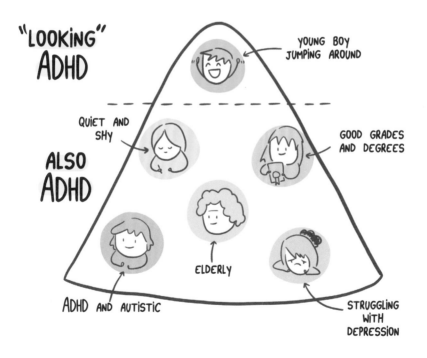

"LOOKING" ADHD

YOUNG BOY JUMPING AROUND

QUIET AND SHY

GOOD GRADES AND DEGREES

ALSO ADHD

ELDERLY

ADHD AND AUTISTIC

STRUGGLING WITH DEPRESSION

ADHD is a
NEURODEVELOPMENTAL DISORDER

A neurodevelopmental disorder is a condition that affects the development of the brain and nervous system. As a result, people with ADHD have a brain that works differently from those without ADHD. It also means that people with ADHD are born with the condition and will have it all their lives.

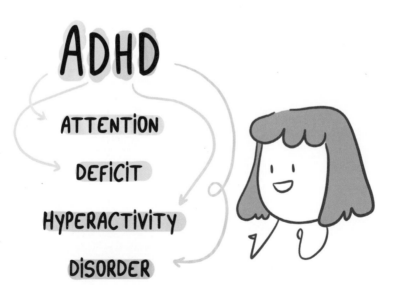

ADHD

ATTENTION

DEFICIT

HYPERACTIVITY

DISORDER

ADHD IS (PROBABLY) CAUSED BY GENETICS

Scientists are still not entirely sure what causes ADHD, but more and more specialists believe that it could be linked to genetics. This could explain why experts believe the chance of inheriting ADHD is around 80 percent. If your family is full of ADHDers, this could be why!

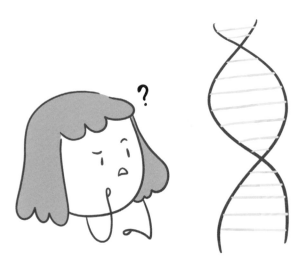

ADHD IS LINKED TO DOPAMINE

Many believe that ADHD could be linked to dopamine. Dopamine is a neurotransmitter, mainly responsible for feelings of pleasure and reward. According to some studies, people with ADHD have lower levels of dopamine. That's why stimulant medications, which increase dopamine levels, are sometimes used to treat ADHD.

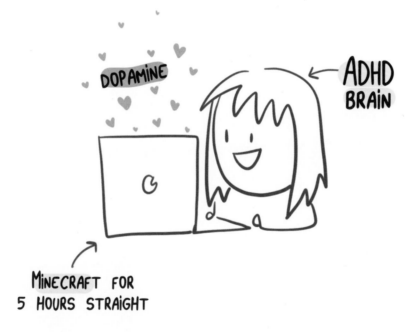

HAVING ADHD MEANS HAVING A DIFFERENT BRAIN

ADHD is a neurodevelopmental disorder, which means that people with ADHD have brains that have developed in a different way to people without ADHD. Even though there have been very few studies carried out on the brains of people with ADHD, in one experiment, scientists were able to identify 79.3 percent of the people who had an ADHD diagnosis just by looking at the structure of their brains.

ADHD BRAINS ARE DIFFERENT

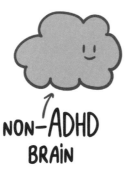

NON-ADHD BRAIN

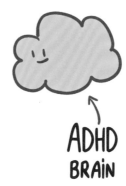

ADHD BRAIN

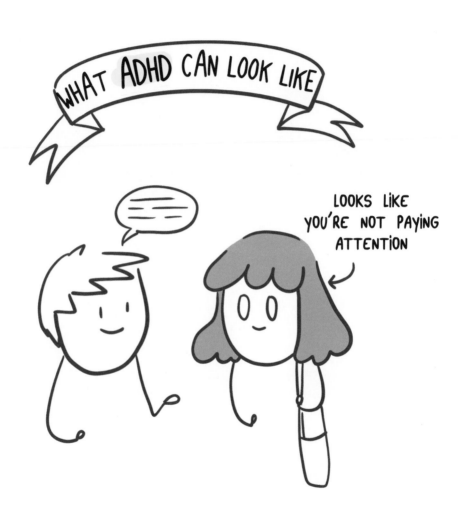

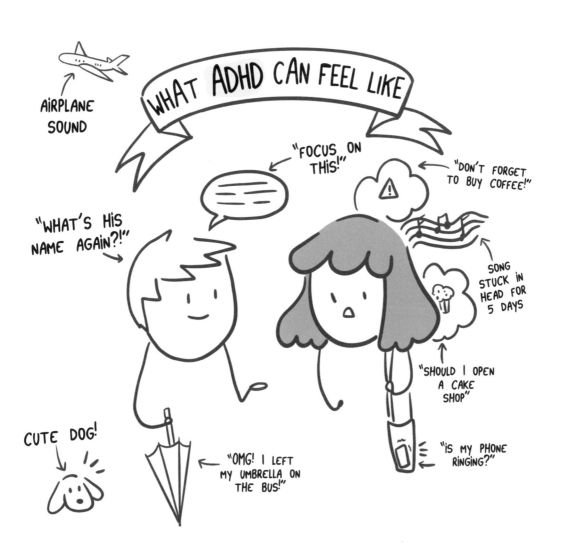

The three types of ADHD

Did you know that people diagnosed with ADHD often experience the condition quite differently from one another? This is because everyone has subjective experiences, but it's also because there are three types of ADHD.

The American Psychiatric Association has identified these as:

- predominantly hyperactive-impulsive
- predominantly inattentive
- combined

Each type has a specific set of symptoms that impact life in various ways. Even if you are diagnosed with one type of ADHD at a point in your life (for example, if you were diagnosed with hyperactive type as a child), it's possible to show symptoms of another type later in life. Many people with ADHD learn to mask hyperactive symptoms growing up and are diagnosed with inattentive type ADHD as adults.

ADHD
HYPERACTIVE TYPE

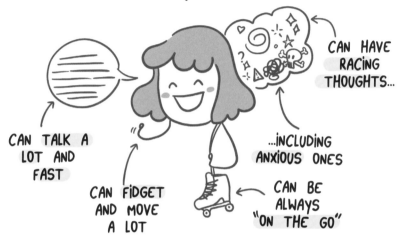

CAN HAVE RACING THOUGHTS...

CAN TALK A LOT AND FAST

...INCLUDING ANXIOUS ONES

CAN FIDGET AND MOVE A LOT

CAN BE ALWAYS "ON THE GO"

Having this type of ADHD means experiencing mainly hyperactive and impulsive symptoms (you'll see examples of symptoms in the next chapter). It doesn't mean you don't struggle with inattention or forgetfulness, but it's less pronounced than in someone with the inattentive or combined types. People with hyperactive type ADHD can be mentally hyperactive, physically hyperactive or both. The predominantly hyperactive-impulsive type is less common among adults, but it's the most common type among preschool children.

ADHD iNATTENTIVE TYPE

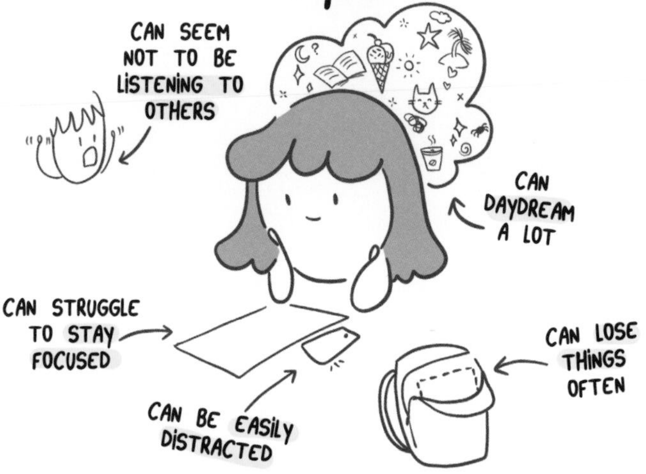

CAN SEEM NOT TO BE LISTENING TO OTHERS

CAN DAYDREAM A LOT

CAN STRUGGLE TO STAY FOCUSED

CAN LOSE THINGS OFTEN

CAN BE EASILY DISTRACTED

People with inattentive ADHD are often called "daydreamers." They mostly struggle with forgetfulness, distraction, and inattention. They may seem a bit "spacey" and lost in their own mind. People with the inattentive type of ADHD usually experience a lower level of physical hyperactivity.

ADHD COMBINED TYPE

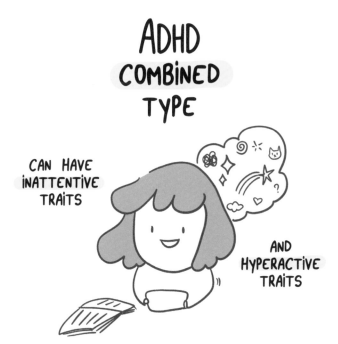

CAN HAVE INATTENTIVE TRAITS

AND HYPERACTIVE TRAITS

People with this type of ADHD can struggle with inattention and forgetfulness, but also with hyperactivity and impulsivity. The intensity of their symptoms can vary and they sometimes mask their hyperactive and impulsive side. Many people diagnosed with ADHD as adults are combined type, with a tendency to experience more mental than physical hyperactivity.

ADHD or ADD?

The term ADD is no longer used in most countries and has been replaced with the acronym ADHD. ADD was previously used to describe individuals with ADHD who did not display many symptoms of hyperactivity in comparison with others. It was replaced with the overall term ADHD by the American Psychiatric Association in 1987.

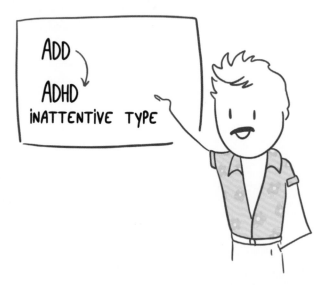

The concept of ADHD subtypes was then introduced in 1994. If you were previously diagnosed with ADD, it's likely that your diagnosis would now be known as ADHD inattentive type.

How common is ADHD?

People are often surprised to know how many people around them have ADHD, but ADHD is not a rare condition, and it has now become more well known and talked about. Adult ADHD has an estimated worldwide prevalence of 2.8 percent, so it's likely that you already know someone who has it.

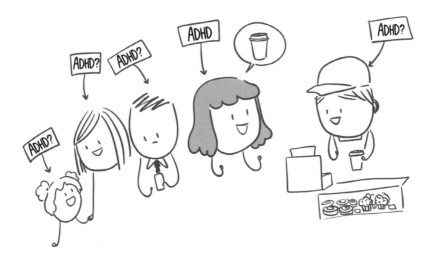

In some studies, the number of people with ADHD in the US is estimated to be as high as 4.4 percent of the adult population—that's close to potentially 15 million people with ADHD in the US alone! However, it's not a figure that's easy to calculate: there are many misdiagnoses, many adults are still undiagnosed, and some countries do not even collect this data.

ADHD misconceptions

"ADHD IS A BOY DISORDER"

I HAVE ADHD

For a long time, ADHD was often associated with the image of a young boy fidgeting, unable to sit still, and throwing tantrums. This is a very outdated and stereotypical view of ADHD, and it's far from the much more complex reality. ADHD affects everyone differently, regardless of gender or age.

ARE YOU SURE? BECAUSE YOU DON'T ACT LIKE MY LITTLE NEPHEW...

"ADHD IS LAZINESS"

I STRUGGLE SO MUCH...

Do people with ADHD struggle with procrastination and have difficulty initiating tasks? Yes. Are they lazy? Certainly not. Most people with ADHD have to try harder than people without ADHD to accomplish the same tasks. It is detrimental to perceive ADHD as laziness, as undiagnosed people will often feel tremendous shame, thinking they are "just lazy." The reality is much more complex than that.

MAYBE YOU SHOULD TRY HARDER?

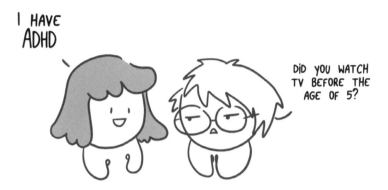

"ADHD IS THE RESULT OF BAD PARENTING"

Too much sugar, too much TV, too many toys... Many people will tell you they believe ADHD results from bad parenting. Even though the causes of ADHD are still not properly understood, we do know that it's something you are born with, and not something you develop because of how you are raised.

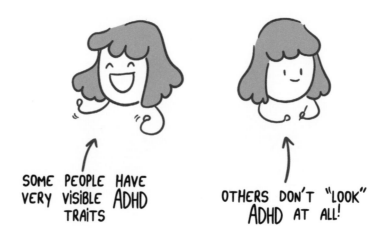

SOME PEOPLE HAVE
VERY VISIBLE ADHD
TRAITS

OTHERS DON'T "LOOK"
ADHD AT ALL!

"ADHD IS OBVIOUS"

This misconception is one of the reasons why so many people are not yet diagnosed. ADHD is not always noticeable (even though it can be!) and most of the time, you can't tell for sure if someone has ADHD or not. That's because all people with ADHD are different and will act and react in their own way. It's also why ADHD is not always easy to diagnose, as we will see in the next chapter.

When it comes to ADHD, many factors are still to be discovered. Even though it's been well researched and we have excellent specialists talking about it, ADHD is still widely misunderstood. I hope this chapter helped you understand more about ADHD, without being too overwhelming. In the next chapter, we'll discover everything you need to know about an ADHD diagnosis! And remember:

ADHD is one of the most common developmental disorders among children.

ADHD brains work differently from non-ADHD brains.

Two people with ADHD can have different experiences.

There are still many misconceptions about ADHD.

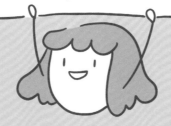

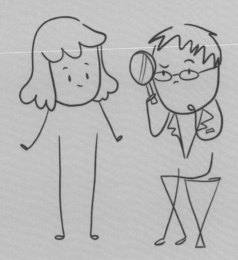

THE ADHD DIAGNOSIS

CHAPTER 2

Who can diagnose ADHD?

ADHD can only officially be diagnosed by a health professional. In most countries psychiatrists are the recognized professionals who conduct official assessments.

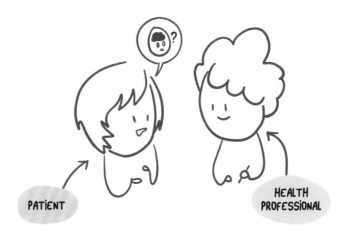

THE PATIENT EXPLAINS THEIR EXPERIENCE
TO THEIR HEALTH PROFESSIONAL

The ADHD assessment

ADHD is diagnosed through a clinical evaluation, where a health professional observes your symptoms. Some countries and professionals offer brain scans or other tests, but this isn't the case everywhere. It's likely that several questionnaires and official lists of symptoms would be used for assessment, such as those found in the latest edition of the *Diagnostic and Statistical Manual of Mental Disorders* (or DSM-5).

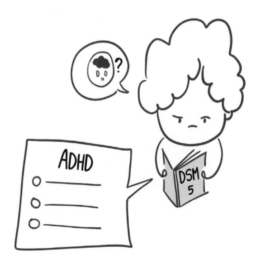

To diagnose you, the professional will need to see that you exhibit most of the symptoms, that they have a negative impact on your life, and that you have experienced the symptoms for longer than a few months.

Symptoms of ADHD

In most countries, you need to experience at least five symptoms of inattention and five symptoms of hyperactivity in order to be diagnosed with ADHD. To be sure that it's not another condition, you must experience these symptoms for more than six months. And they need to impact at least two areas of your life, for example, work and relationships.

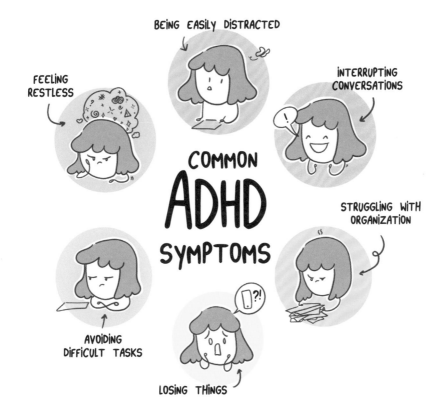

BEING EASILY DISTRACTED

INTERRUPTING CONVERSATIONS

FEELING RESTLESS

COMMON
ADHD
SYMPTOMS

STRUGGLING WITH ORGANIZATION

AVOIDING DIFFICULT TASKS

LOSING THINGS

INATTENTIVE SYMPTOMS

Experiencing forgetfulness and distractibility, like losing your phone, keys, and wallet all the time, or zoning out when someone is talking to you, are a major part of inattentive symptoms. But remember that many people with ADHD develop strategies to hide or overcompensate for these traits. That's why, for example, you might never lose your belongings, but maybe you are constantly checking that you have them because you are afraid of losing them.

Here are some inattentive symptoms:

- Being easily distracted
- Having difficulties with organization
- Struggling to focus your attention
- Making frequent mistakes
- Difficulty with following instructions

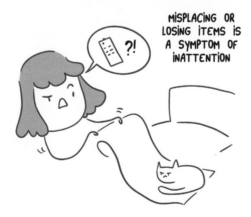

MISPLACING OR LOSING ITEMS IS A SYMPTOM OF INATTENTION

HYPERACTIVE-IMPULSIVE SYMPTOMS

ADHD hyperactivity is much more than just having trouble staying seated for long periods of time. Mental hyperactivity, for example, might cause you to struggle to fall asleep at night because of racing thoughts. You may interrupt people during conversations, tend to impulse buy, or even fidget. All these things can be symptoms of hyperactivity and impulsivity.

Here are some hyperactive symptoms:
- Fidgeting
- Feeling restless
- Having difficulty relaxing
- Talking a lot and very quickly
- Interrupting others during conversations

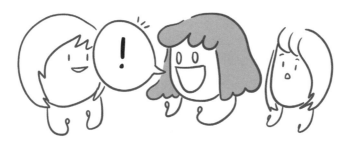

INTERRUPTING PEOPLE DURING CONVERSATIONS
IS A SYMPTOM OF IMPULSIVITY

UNOFFICIAL SYMPTOMS

Many people with ADHD experience traits that are not on the official list of symptoms. Even though they may not form part of the official ADHD criteria, they are often part of the ADHD experience. These can be issues like struggling with perception of time, difficulty managing emotions, feeling rejection very strongly, being able to focus on specific things intensely, or being extremely sensitive to sensory input.

Here are some unofficial symptoms:
- Struggling with sleep
- Having sensory issues, such as sensitivity to noise, textures, or foods
- Being very sensitive to rejection or criticism
- Struggling with time awareness
- Hyperfocusing on interesting things

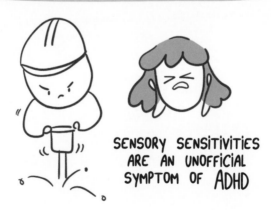

SENSORY SENSITIVITIES ARE AN UNOFFICIAL SYMPTOM OF ADHD

HOW ADHD CAN AFFECT EMOTIONS

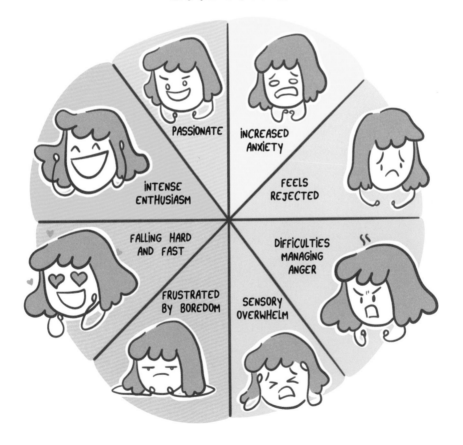

Why are so many people diagnosed with ADHD later in life?

More and more adults are being diagnosed with ADHD later in life. That's because we now know that this disorder can present itself more subtly than was previously understood.

In recent years, many people with ADHD have chosen to talk openly about their diagnosis, which has helped to remove some of the stigma around the condition. But there are still many factors that prevent adults from being diagnosed.

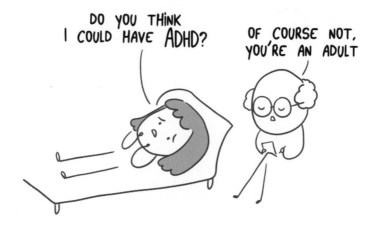

COST OF DIAGNOSIS

In many countries, an ADHD assessment made by a professional can cost a lot of money. When you add in the fact that people with ADHD often struggle with employment and money management issues, it's clear that the cost of diagnosis can be a reason why some adults are still living with undiagnosed ADHD today.

LONG WAITING LIST

Even if you live in a country with free public healthcare, the demand for assessment is often so high that waiting lists are incredibly long. It's common to hear people from these countries say they are on a two-year waiting list to be assessed.

FEAR OF BEING DISMISSED

Many adults are not ready to start their ADHD diagnosis journey, because they dread being dismissed if they talk about their situation with a health professional. Unfortunately, sometimes it happens. If a health professional is telling you that you don't have ADHD, but they haven't taken the time to evaluate this properly, it's a good idea to seek a second opinion.

Related disorders

Because ADHD symptoms are sometimes similar to symptoms of other disorders, it can be hard for people with ADHD to get a diagnosis for another condition, such as anxiety or depression. For example, having trouble focusing can also be a symptom of depression, and impulsive behavior can also be a feature of borderline personality disorder (BPD). If your diagnosis doesn't feel right, ask for a second opinion or speak to friends and family members about how you are feeling.

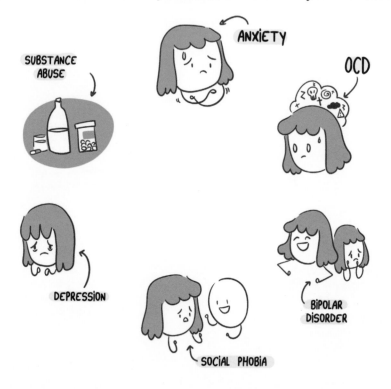

Getting an ADHD diagnosis is not always easy. This is in part because ADHD is complex and can impact people differently, but also because other mental health conditions can hide ADHD symptoms. Even though awareness of ADHD has increased, many people, including some mental health professionals, still have a very stereotypical view of it. I hope things will change in the coming years, so that everyone wondering if they have ADHD can quickly get the answers they deserve. In the next chapter, we will look at what to do with these answers when you finally receive them. And remember:

An ADHD diagnosis must come from a healthcare professional.

ADHD can sometimes be misdiagnosed or overlooked, especially if you don't fit the stereotype.

Symptoms of ADHD can vary from one person to another.

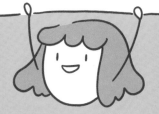

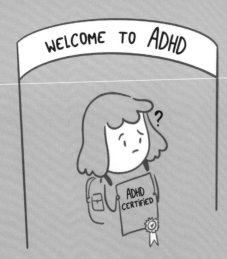

WELCOME TO ADHD

ADHD CERTIFIED

WHAT HAPPENS AFTER AN ADHD DIAGNOSIS?

CHAPTER 3

Managing emotions after an ADHD diagnosis

It's normal to feel a lot of different emotions after an ADHD diagnosis. It's a big step and many people need time to adjust emotionally. When I was diagnosed with ADHD at the age of 29, I felt instant relief. I finally had an answer to the question I had always asked myself: "What's wrong with me?" The answer was that nothing was wrong. I was just different.

But this pleasant feeling of relief was soon replaced by other emotions, like sadness, anger, and confusion. I remember that the months that followed my diagnosis were complicated, and I experienced many strong and conflicting emotions, which I wasn't prepared for.

MANY PEOPLE DOUBT THEIR ADHD DIAGNOSIS ONCE THEY FINALLY GET IT. IF YOU DO, TOO, YOU ARE NOT ALONE

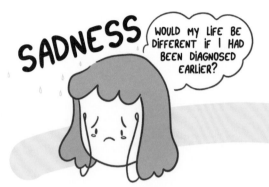

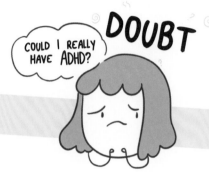

It's quite normal to feel sad after your ADHD diagnosis. I felt extremely downhearted for some weeks after I received mine. Depending on your age, you might feel like you have missed out on part of your life. You could be thinking that you might have done things differently if you had known. You might reflect and see how your undiagnosed ADHD has impacted your career, love life, and self-esteem. It's OK to feel like you are grieving. Take your time and ask for help if it's too much to go through alone.

Many people seek an assessment for ADHD because they are confused or uncertain about their symptoms. Unfortunately, even after being formally diagnosed with ADHD, some doubt that the diagnosis is correct; they may feel like an imposter or struggle to accept that they have ADHD. I felt like this for weeks after my diagnosis. If you have similar feelings, it's a good idea to talk to someone about them. And remember that you are allowed to ask for a second opinion if something feels "off" about your diagnosis.

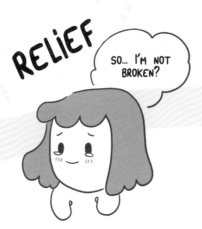

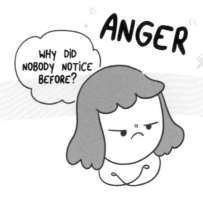

Some people feel that a considerable weight is lifted when they get their ADHD diagnosis. That's how I felt when my psychiatrist told me the result of my assessment. I left the appointment with a big smile on my face. When you spend years thinking "What's wrong with me?" without finding any answers, having a label to put to your struggles can be a relief. If you are experiencing this, enjoy it and embrace the peace of mind this new information is offering you.

If you are filled with rage and anger after getting your ADHD diagnosis, you are not alone. Emotional reactions to diagnosis can be extreme, especially if it happens later in life. I definitely felt this way. You may ask yourself why nobody noticed that you may have had a condition that required help. You might be angry if you had to wait a long time to get assessed, thinking that you've lost precious months or years. This emotional reaction is normal, and you should try to accept the feelings of anger as they arise, because they are justified.

Talking about your diagnosis

If you just got your ADHD diagnosis, it's normal to want to talk about it with your friends and family. But you may also want to keep it to yourself. Here are a few tips to help you share information with the people around you.

I HAVE SOMETHING TO TELL YOU...

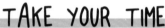

TAKE YOUR TIME

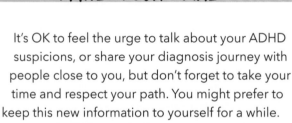

It's OK to feel the urge to talk about your ADHD suspicions, or share your diagnosis journey with people close to you, but don't forget to take your time and respect your path. You might prefer to keep this new information to yourself for a while. A diagnosis of ADHD can feel very private, and you are allowed to be discreet about it.

- Journaling can help you process your emotions regarding your diagnosis before you start talking about it.
- Sharing your concerns with a health professional can help you prepare before talking to your friends and family.

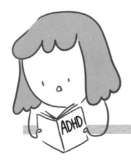

LEARN A LOT

ADHD is a complex condition. The more you learn about it, the better you will be able to explain the details to others. When you get your diagnosis, it is possible that the health professional conducting the assessment won't give you much information about ADHD. I didn't receive much explanation when I got mine. But learning about ADHD after your diagnosis will allow you to do something very important: understand yourself.

- Joining an online forum about ADHD can help you share your experience with others and understand how some of your behaviors are linked to ADHD.
- Reading books (like this one!) or listening to a podcast are also great ways to learn about the complexities of your brain.
- Learning about ADHD will help you better explain your symptoms to your friends and family. It could also give you some ideas about how they can support you.

HOW TO RESPOND TO NEGATIVITY

You will sometimes face negative reactions if you talk about your ADHD diagnosis. It's unfortunate, but some people will need a bit more time to be able to listen to you. It can also be an excellent opportunity to change some minds about the reality of ADHD, but remember that some people might not be able or willing to understand what you are experiencing.

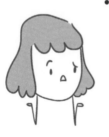

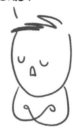

- Older people can have trouble understanding ADHD. They might come from a generation where mental health was not an easy thing to talk about. So before talking about it to your grandmother or other family members, be prepared to face some surprising comments (trust me, I've been there!).

- If you face adverse reactions when you decide to talk about your diagnosis, know that you don't have to fight for your cause if you don't want to. When people are open about their diagnoses, it can be a great way to raise awareness of ADHD. But if you don't feel able to discuss it in this way, that's OK too. You don't have to expend energy trying to change the mind of someone who isn't open to it.

Finding support

Getting a diagnosis is just the start of your journey. Now that you have this new information about yourself, it's time to find solutions and accommodations to make your life easier.

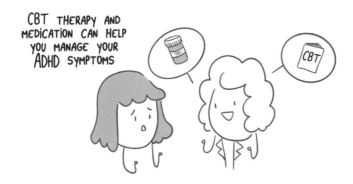

FIND THE RIGHT THERAPEUTIC APPROACH

ADHD is not curable. But there are many things you can try to limit the negative impacts of ADHD symptoms on your life. Therapeutic approaches like cognitive behavioral therapy (CBT) might help you reduce impulsivity and improve emotional stability. Medication is also an interesting solution that may be worth trying. Talk to your mental health professional to find the right therapeutic path for you.

TAKING MEDICATION FOR ADHD?

The decision whether or not to take medication for ADHD is deeply personal. Some people find it difficult to tolerate the side effects (like loss of appetite, sleep difficulties, or headaches), while others will find medication extremely beneficial. Whichever path you choose, remember that this decision is entirely yours. I know people who don't feel like they need medication at all and others who are thriving under treatment with medication. We should all respect each other's choices.

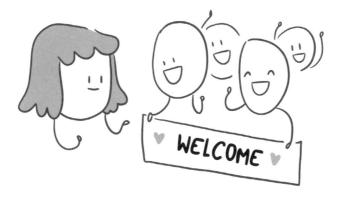

FINDING A COMMUNITY OF PEOPLE WITH
ADHD WILL HELP YOU FEEL LESS LONELY

JOIN COMMUNITIES

If you have recently been diagnosed with ADHD, there are online communities you can join that offer support if you feel afraid to talk about your ADHD diagnosis with friends and family. You could also discover new ideas to help solve some of your daily challenges. Most of all, you may see that although people with ADHD are all different, you can relate to many of their struggles and experiences. With time, you might even make new friends!

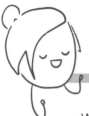
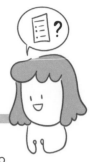

Ask for Accommodations

Whether you are studying or working, ADHD is likely to have an impact on your daily life and productivity. If you struggle, don't be afraid to ask for accommodations. These don't have to be complicated to help you feel more supported and more productive. Here are some ideas for accommodations that might help.

BEING SUPPORTED BY A KIND TEAM

Meeting regularly with a co-worker to increase accountability

Using emojis in messages to help convey emotions and avoid misunderstandings

Having regular check-ins to measure the impact of accommodations

WORKING IN AN ADAPTED ENVIRONMENT

Having a standing desk

Being able to work in a quiet room

Having access to a whiteboard to use visualization techniques

COMMUNICATING EFFICIENTLY

Recording meetings instead of taking notes

Allowing time for focus without interruptions (email, messages, etc.)

Having written instructions instead of verbal ones

Getting an official ADHD diagnosis is the end of your diagnosis journey (which can be pretty long). But it's also the start of a new journey. Whether it's an easy or a difficult start, down the road, this new information will help you to understand yourself better and advocate for your needs. In the next chapter, you will discover words and expressions that can help you describe and share your experiences. And remember:

Experiencing strong and confusing emotions after an ADHD diagnosis is normal.

You can share your ADHD diagnosis or keep it private. It is your choice.

Once you are diagnosed with ADHD, there are many ways to find support.

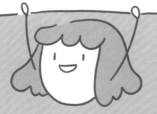

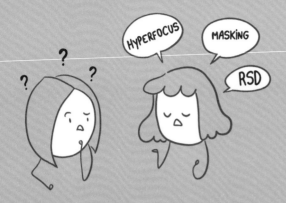

ADHD GLOSSARY

CHAPTER 4

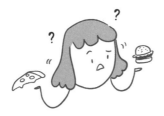

AnAlysis pAralysis

ADHD often impacts your ability to make decisions quickly. It's because making decisions, even small ones (like deciding what to have for dinner), is a complex act that requires different skills. To make a decision, you need to consider the various options, remember them, and compare them. If you add time pressure, it's not hard to imagine how we can "get stuck" and feel like it's almost impossible to make a decision. And that's how you can end up eating peanut butter from the jar for dinner.

Anxiety

Adults with ADHD are 2.5 times more likely to struggle with anxiety than adults without ADHD. Often, ADHD symptoms and the symptoms of generalized anxiety disorder, such as feeling restless, having difficulty concentrating, and being fearful or worried, can be confused, even for mental health professionals. Do you constantly worry because you suffer from anxiety, or is anxiety a consequence of your unmanaged ADHD symptoms? If you have the slightest doubt, getting a proper assessment for anxiety as someone with ADHD is always a good idea.

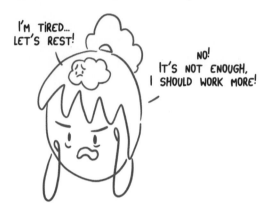

SOMETIMES, PEOPLE WITH **ADHD** EVEN STRUGGLE TO REST BECAUSE THEY ARE TERRIFIED OF LOOKING "LAZY"

I'M TIRED... LET'S REST!

NO! IT'S NOT ENOUGH, I SHOULD WORK MORE!

BURNOUT

It's common for people with ADHD to experience burnout. You may overcompensate at work, or mask with friends and family so they don't notice you zoning out. Managing your symptoms is not easy and can lead to exhaustion and burnout. Having to deal with yet another burnout at 29 made me realize something was not right, and ultimately led to me seeking an ADHD assessment.

OVERCOMPENSATION

As we go through life with ADHD, we tend to develop habits and skills to compensate for some of our symptoms. For example, many people with ADHD struggle with time awareness and will often be late for meetings with friends or professional events. To try and avoid this, some people with ADHD will develop the habit of always being early. This kind of overcompensation can create new issues. You can quickly develop anxiety if you constantly try to anticipate the problems your ADHD traits could cause (like being unable to send an email unless you've read it at least ten times).

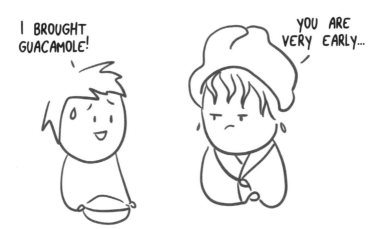

EMOTIONAL DYSREGULATION

OTHER PEOPLE

ME

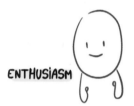

ENTHUSIASM

Emotional dysregulation is an emotional reaction that does not fall within the traditionally accepted range. Even though it's not part of the official diagnosis criteria, many think it's an overlooked symptom of ADHD.

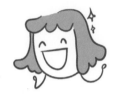

SADNESS

Do you often struggle to cool down after feelings of anger? Do you think your enthusiasm is "over the top" when you feel passionate about a topic? Do you feel sad more easily than others? Well, you are not alone.

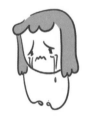

ANGER

When emotional dysregulation is not identified, it can lead to questions like "Why did I react like that?" or "Why am I always too much?"

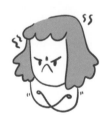

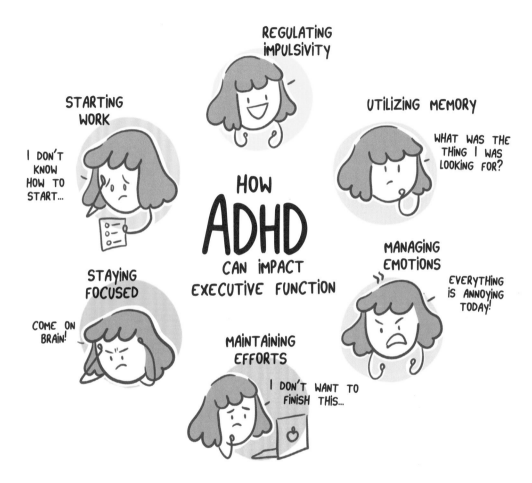

EXECUTIVE FUNCTIONS

Executive functions allow us to think before we act, imagine scenarios, resist temptations, and stay focused. ADHD impacts executive functioning and may be why you struggle to remember a phone number, have trouble paying attention, or interrupt people while they are talking. This executive dysfunction may impact your professional or personal life, but it can be improved by doing various exercises and activities, such as memory games and playing music.

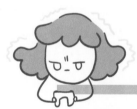

HYPERFOCUS

Hyperfocus describes a highly focused state of attention. It feels like you are in a bubble. You may even lose track of time, fail to notice people around you, and even ignore your own needs and forget to drink, eat, or take a bathroom break. Needless to say, when you finally exit this state of hyperfocus you could be exhausted, hungry, and uncomfortable!

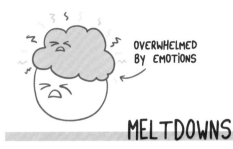

MELTDOWNS

People with ADHD experience meltdowns because they struggle to regulate feelings of frustration, anger, or overwhelm. Sensory overload may also cause these extreme emotional reactions. I felt ashamed of my meltdowns for most of my adult life. I now understand my triggers and warning signs, so I can rest and take a break.

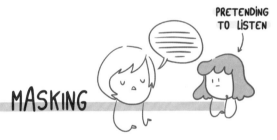

MASKING

Masking means hiding your traits in order to appear "normal." The tendency to hide ADHD behavior varies greatly from person to person. Some are so good at it (knowingly or not) that they are even misdiagnosed with another condition, or remain undiagnosed with ADHD. That's why it's important to mention to the person assessing you that you are adapting and camouflaging your behavior during an ADHD assessment.

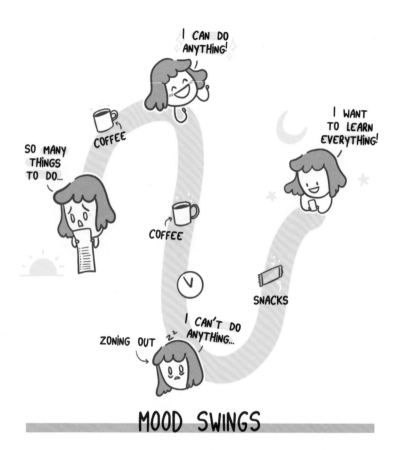

MOOD SWINGS

Because people with ADHD often experience emotional dysregulation, their days can be punctuated by mood swings. Mixed with impulsivity, our difficulty moderating our emotions may lead to us experiencing various moods in a day. From feeling anxious about your to-do list when you wake up to having a burst of enthusiasm when you talk about your new project with a friend, going through all these emotions is pretty tiring. No wonder you suddenly feel exhausted in the middle of the day!

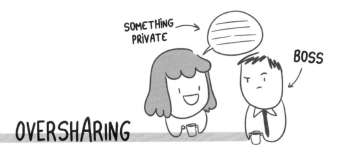

OVERSHARING

Because of their impulsivity, many people with ADHD tend to share more than they initially wanted to. It's OK to share personal things if you want to, but oversharing can sometimes lead to regret. It can even make you feel shameful after social situations where you had trouble managing your impulsivity. It's not fun when you realize that you've been boring your boss by talking about your nicknames for your cat for the past 15 minutes!

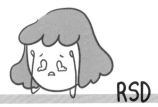

RSD

RSD, or rejection sensitive dysphoria, is used in the ADHD community to describe the extreme sensitivity to rejection that some people with ADHD can struggle with. People who experience RSD describe the experience of feeling rejected or criticized as excruciating pain. It's not a medical diagnosis, but some mental health professionals think it helps to describe the emotional dysregulation of people with ADHD.

THE ADHD TAX

People with ADHD face a variety of challenges daily.
Sometimes these struggles end up costing us money.
That's what the ADHD community calls the ADHD tax. It can
be things like letting food perish in your fridge, getting fines
because you forgot to take back books to the library, or
failing to return clothes or items on time. My worst ADHD tax
was when I noticed I was still paying for a gym membership
years after I had moved to another city!

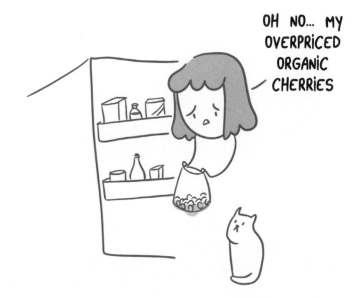

OH NO... MY
OVERPRICED
ORGANIC
CHERRIES

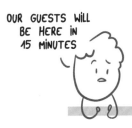

OUR GUESTS WILL BE HERE IN 15 MINUTES

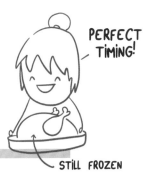

PERFECT TIMING!

STILL FROZEN

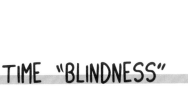

TIME "BLINDNESS"

Time "blindness" is an expression used in the ADHD community to describe a lack of awareness of time. People with ADHD often report struggling with time management. Their "time horizon," meaning how far they can project their thoughts into the future, often feels shorter than it does for neurotypical people. And because of hyperfocus, people with ADHD can also get stuck in "interest bubbles" and lose track of time, for example, being late to work because of a fascinating article or video.

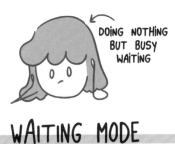

DOING NOTHING BUT BUSY WAITING

WAITING MODE

People with ADHD can often feel stuck waiting. For example, if you have an appointment at 3 p.m., you might feel like you can't focus on anything else that day because anticipating the appointment takes up a huge part of your mind.

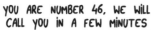

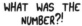

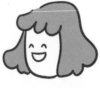

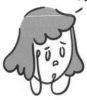

WORKING MEMORY

Working memory is a cognitive skill that helps our brain retain information temporarily, such as what you wanted to say during a conversation or where you parked your car. For many people with ADHD, our working memory is weaker or less developed because of our ADHD symptoms. It can be frustrating to deal with it when you rely on your brain to pay attention and retain pieces of information.

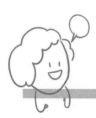

ZONING OUT

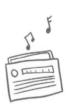

Zoning out is the feeling of not being conscious of what's happening around you when you are in the middle of a conversation. It happens to everyone once in a while. But for people with ADHD, it can happen several times per day. And it can be a bit tricky to explain to the person you're talking with that you didn't quite hear what they said for the last two minutes.

In this chapter, we covered some of the basic terms people in the ADHD community use to describe their symptoms. Having the right words to describe our life with ADHD is crucial to being able to understand and explain what we are going through every day.

In the next part of the book, I'll take you along with me in a day with ADHD. You'll see how the way our brain works can have an impact on every single aspect of our daily lives. And remember:

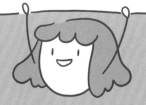

The fact that these phrases exist is proof that you are not the only one experiencing them.

This glossary is not exhaustive, as the ADHD community is always creating new ways to depict the challenges we face.

PART 2

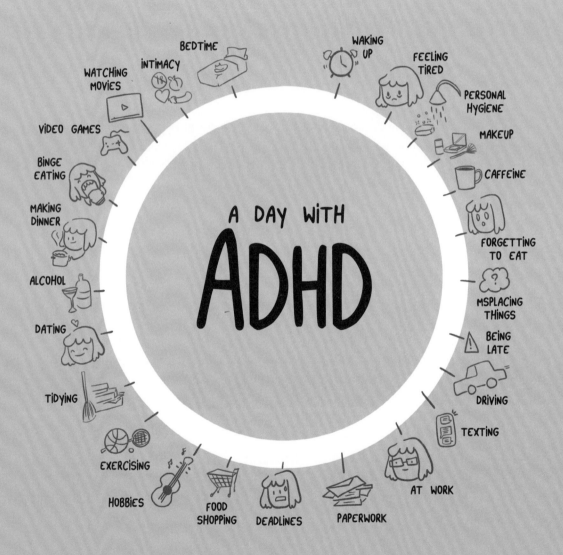

What is it like to live with ADHD? That's the question I asked myself many times before and after my diagnosis. I knew the theory, but I wanted to see concrete examples of how it affected my daily life; my real life. From the moment you wake up, to the moment you (struggle to) fall asleep, ADHD symptoms are shaping your day. Let's try to understand how ADHD impacts you, to help you make peace with yourself and find solutions.

A DAY WITH ADHD

Waking up

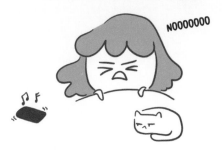

STRUGGLING TO GET OUT OF BED
IS A UNIVERSAL EXPERIENCE.
BUT IT CAN BE EVEN HARDER
FOR PEOPLE WITH ADHD

NOOOOOOO

MY EXPERIENCE

I struggle to get out of bed almost every morning. No matter
what I do, it takes me hours to get out of my warm bed.
As I often fall asleep late (we'll talk about that later), I need
a moment to feel fully awake. But that's when trouble arises.
To help me wake up, I get on my phone, which opens the
door to an infinite number of distractions. That's why I
can be late for anything, even if I miraculously manage to
wake up on time!

BECAUSE THEY CAN TEND TO GO TO BED LATE...

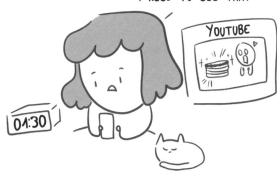

BECAUSE THEY STRUGGLE TO FALL ASLEEP QUICKLY...

BECAUSE THEY FEEL OVERWHLEMED BY THE THINGS THEY HAVE TO DO...

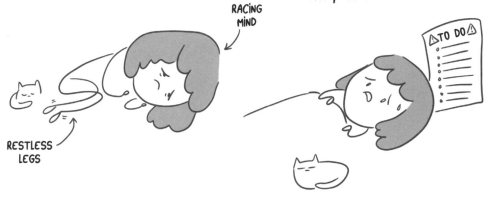

OR THEY ARE EASILY DISTRACTED...

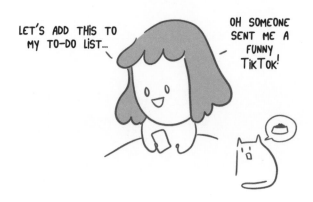

UNTIL THEY REALIZE THEY ARE GOING TO BE LATE!

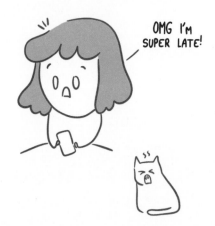

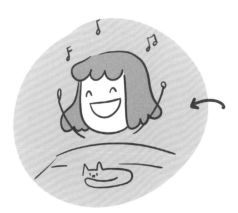

When I feel like I need a special boost to get out of bed, I play upbeat music. It usually does the trick.

If I know I have an important appointment the next day, I put my phone far away from my bed, so I don't have the temptation to scroll for hours the following morning.

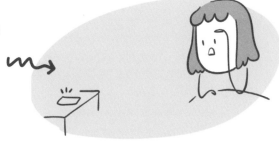

Always feeling tired

MANY PEOPLE THiNK THAT PEOPLE WiTH ADHD ALWAYS HAVE A LOT OF ENERGY...

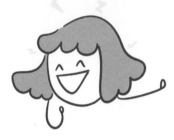

MY EXPERIENCE

I think the hyperactivity aspect of ADHD can sometimes be misleading. I'm definitely hyperactive (at least mentally!), but I'm also hyper-tired. Having to deal with my symptoms and their consequences is exhausting. Because I'm always trying to remember things and keep my head above water, I often don't have the energy to do the things I enjoy doing.

BUT DID YOU KNOW THAT MANY
PEOPLE WITH ADHD ACTUALLY
FEEL TIRED ALL THE TIME?

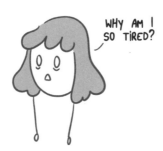

WHY AM I
SO TIRED?

THIS TIREDNESS CAN
BE CAUSED BY...

...OR BY SLEEP STRUGGLES THAT
OFTEN COME WITH ADHD...

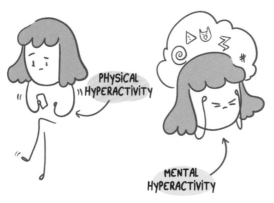

PHYSICAL
HYPERACTIVITY

MENTAL
HYPERACTIVITY

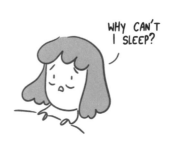

WHY CAN'T
I SLEEP?

...OR BECAUSE OF SENSORY OVERLOADS

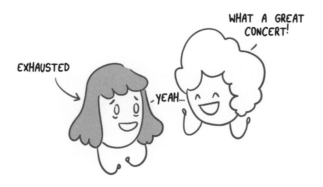

EXHAUSTED

YEAH...

WHAT A GREAT CONCERT!

...OR BECAUSE OF CONDITIONS THAT OFTEN CO-OCCUR WITH ADHD...

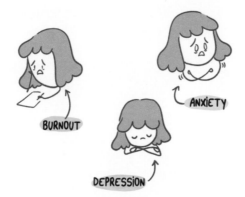

BURNOUT

DEPRESSION

ANXIETY

IF YOU HAVE ADHD AND ARE TIRED ALL THE TIME, IT CAN COME FROM MANY DIFFERENT THINGS...

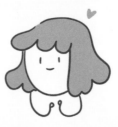

...IN ANY CASE, IT'S ALWAYS BEST TO TALK TO YOUR HEALTH PROFESSIONAL TO FIND A SOLUTION

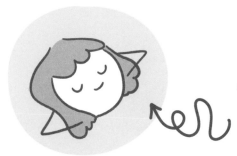

I'm working on taking rest more seriously. Like many people with ADHD, I tend to forget to relax and unwind. I struggle with mindfulness and meditation, but I enjoy simple things like taking a bath or listening to calming music.

Feeling extremely tired all the time is not normal. If you feel something is wrong with you, consult your doctor. I was in this situation once, and I'm glad I took my health seriously, as I got the proper treatment for the issue I was facing.

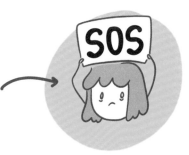

Personal hygiene

DID YOU KNOW THAT PEOPLE WITH ADHD CAN STRUGGLE WITH PERSONAL HYGIENE?

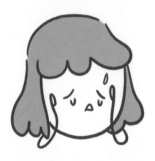

MY EXPERIENCE

Before my diagnosis, I never would have guessed that ADHD could cause some of the struggles I had with personal hygiene. These challenges are invisible to others, but they brought me a lot of shame throughout my life. For example, I often forget to brush my teeth, and I can't count the number of days I have been left with zero clean clothes because I forgot to dry the clothes I washed the day before.

IT'S BECAUSE OUR ABILITY TO MAINTAIN GOOD PERSONAL HYGIENE CAN BE IMPACTED BY ADHD SYMPTOMS...

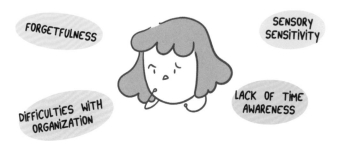

FORGETFULNESS

SENSORY SENSITIVITY

DIFFICULTIES WITH ORGANIZATION

LACK OF TIME AWARENESS

LIKE STRUGGLING TO PLAN WHEN TO WASH YOUR HAIR...

...OR NOT NOTICING YOUR CLOTHES ARE NOT THAT CLEAN...

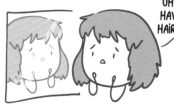

OH NO, I SHOULD HAVE WASHED MY HAIR THIS MORNING!

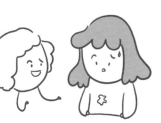

IS THAT MUSTARD?

STRUGGLING WiTH SHOWERING BECAUSE OF SENSORY SENSiTiViTY...

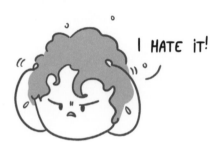

...OR FORGETTING TO BRUSH YOUR TEETH

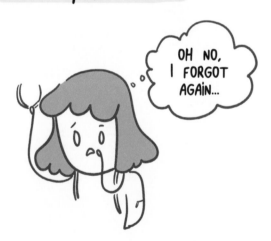

MY ADVICE

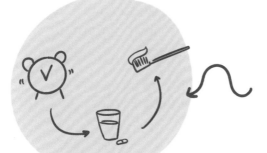

I always stack waking up, taking medication, and brushing my teeth together to avoid forgetting in the morning. You'll learn more about habit stacking in the next part of the book.

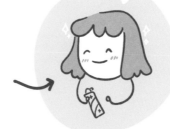

I often procrastinate on washing my hair as I hate the feeling of it. Always having dry shampoo on hand is a must for me.

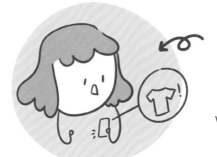

I set a reminder on my phone as soon as I start the washing machine. If I don't, I'm sure to forget, and I'll end up finding wet clothes in my washing machine the next time I need to use it!

Makeup

ADHD CAN IMPACT EVERY ASPECT OF YOUR LIFE, INCLUDING YOUR RELATIONSHIP WITH MAKEUP

LIKE BEING SUPER LATE BUT SINCERELY BELIEVING YOU STILL HAVE TIME TO PUT ON A FULL FACE OF MAKEUP

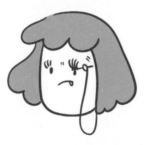

MY EXPERIENCE

Sometimes I love makeup, and I'll spend long minutes doing a full face of it (even though I'm already late), and the next day I'll be happy with just some lip balm. Most of the time, though, I'm too late to take the time to do my makeup correctly, and I throw things around and get it done in five minutes.

FIXATING FOR HOURS ON
RANDOM MAKEUP VIDEOS...

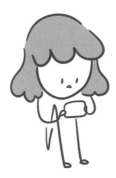

MAKING A HUGE MESS
WHEN GETTING READY...

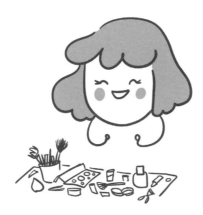

RUINING YOUR MAKEUP BECAUSE
YOU CAN'T STOP TOUCHING
AND RUBBING YOUR FACE...

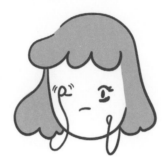

OR HAVING ONLY
TWO MAKEUP MOODS...

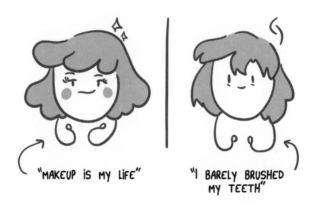

"MAKEUP IS MY LIFE"   "I BARELY BRUSHED
                                MY TEETH"

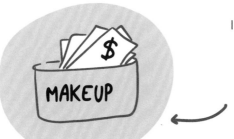

Makeup is one of the things
I tend to impulse buy the most.
But instead of just avoiding
spending money on it, I set
a realistic monthly budget
to still enjoy myself without
too much frustration.

To avoid running late when
I get ready, I timed my "casual"
makeup routine, so now
I know how long I need to be
fully prepared for the day.

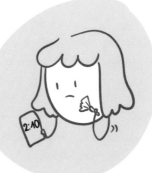

Caffeine

DID YOU KNOW THAT COFFEE CAN AFFECT PEOPLE WITH ADHD DIFFERENTLY?

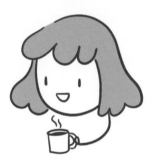

MY EXPERIENCE

I have a love/hate relationship with coffee. Caffeine can help me get stuff done and give me the courage to start some of the most daunting tasks on my to-do list. But too much of it can also seriously exacerbate my mental hyperactivity, even turning it into full-blown anxiety. I've used coffee and tea as stimulants for self-medication for years, and it's now challenging to go without caffeine.

SOME PEOPLE WITH **ADHD** AVOID COFFEE AT ALL COSTS AS IT CAN INCREASE HYPERACTIVITY...

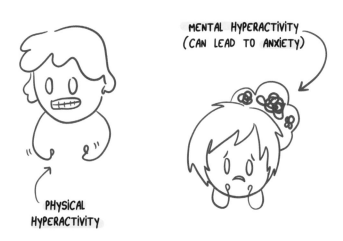

MENTAL HYPERACTIVITY (CAN LEAD TO ANXIETY)

PHYSICAL HYPERACTIVITY

FOR OTHERS, COFFEE CAN HAVE THE OPPOSITE EFFECT AND HELPS THEM RELAX...

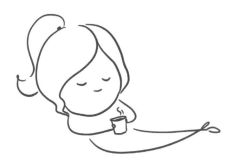

MANY ADULTS WHO ARE UNAWARE OF THEIR ADHD RELY STRONGLY ON COFFEE TO HELP THEM FOCUS

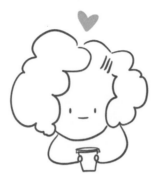

IN SOME CASES, THEY CAN DEVELOP AN EXTREME NEED FOR COFFEE...

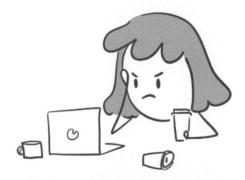

...AND END UP CONSUMING LARGE AMOUNTS OF CAFFEINE

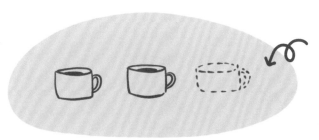

Seeing how my sleep quality and general mental health improved with less caffeine helped me cut down. Even just one cup less per day or switching to decaf after lunch can have a significant impact!

When I feel like I need to go easy on coffee, I try replacing it with lower-caffeine drinks like green tea or hot chocolate, and eating dark chocolate or cacao nibs for a caffeine boost.

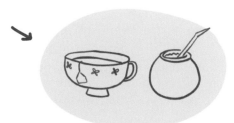

Forgetting to eat

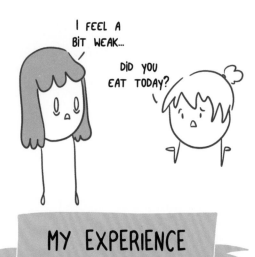

IT'S QUITE COMMON FOR PEOPLE WITH ADHD TO FORGET TO EAT

I FEEL A BIT WEAK...

DID YOU EAT TODAY?

MY EXPERIENCE

I often forget to eat. Sometimes I'm hyperfocusing on something and I completely lose track of time until my stomach starts to growl loudly (of course, it always happens during meetings!). Sometimes my day is so disorganized that I can't find a moment to eat anything. The issue is that when I forget to eat, some of my ADHD traits, like zoning out, get worse. That's why I now prioritize having at least two proper meals every day.

WE CAN HYPERFOCUS SO HARD
ON SOMETHING THAT WE JUST
FORGET ABOUT EVERYTHING ELSE

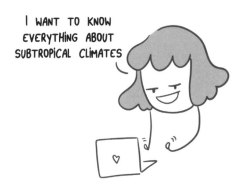

OUR STRUGGLES WITH ORGANIZATION
CAN ALSO MAKE IT A BIT DIFFICULT
TO EAT REGULARLY...

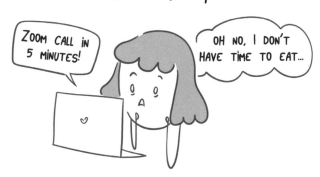

WE ALSO TEND TO STRUGGLE WITH TIME
AWARENESS, WHICH CAN MAKE IT DIFFICULT
TO KEEP TRACK OF MEAL TIMES

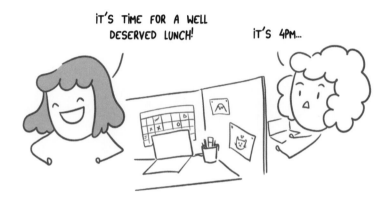

AND ADHD MEDS CAN HAVE THE
TENDENCY TO REDUCE OUR APPETITE...

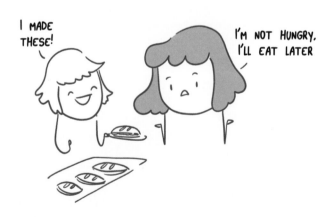

MY ADVICE

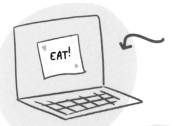

It may sound weird, but I sometimes set reminders on my phone that just say, "Don't forget to eat."

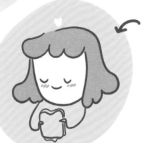

I accept that keeping myself fed means I often have to choose convenient options. A cheese sandwich for lunch might not be Pinterest-worthy, but if it's the only thing I manage to make, it's good enough for me!

When I noticed that my eating habits were getting too chaotic, I consulted a nutritionist who helped me create a meal plan based on my needs.

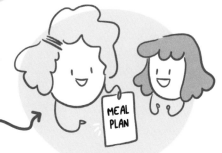

Misplacing things

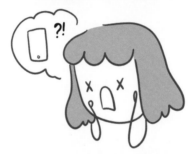

ONE OF THE INATTENTIVE SYMPTOMS OF ADHD IS LOSING STUFF...

MY EXPERIENCE

I tend to be super careful with my belongings when I'm outside of my house, so I rarely lose things. But I misplace stuff all the time. I spend hours every week looking for my glasses, the TV remote, my phone, and kitchen utensils, and I feel as though I am always looking for something. It's exhausting, especially when you notice that the phone you've spent 30 minutes looking for is in your hand!

...THAT'S WHY SOME PEOPLE WITH ADHD COMPENSATE BY BEING VERY CAREFUL WITH THEIR BELONGINGS

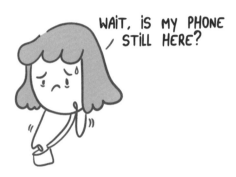

WAIT, IS MY PHONE STILL HERE?

BUT IT DOESN'T MEAN THEY DON'T STRUGGLE WITH MISPLACING STUFF ALL THE TIME

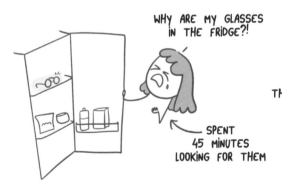

WHY ARE MY GLASSES IN THE FRIDGE?!

SPENT 45 MINUTES LOOKING FOR THEM

SOME PEOPLE WITH ADHD SPEND HOURS EACH DAY LOOKING FOR THINGS

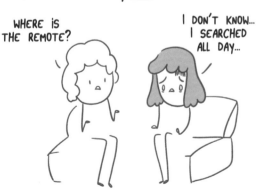

WHERE IS THE REMOTE?

I DON'T KNOW... I SEARCHED ALL DAY...

...ESPECIALLY WHEN OTHER
PEOPLE DON'T UNDERSTAND...

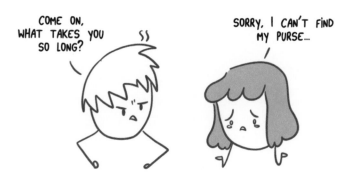

IT CAN BE
MENTALLY EXHAUSTING...

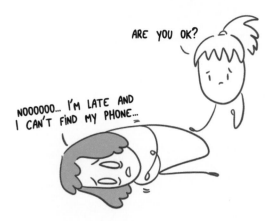

MY ADVICE

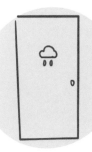

I bought a magnetic key holder for my front door, and I can't tell you how glad I am that I did! Having a specific spot for each thing definitely helps me misplace items less often.

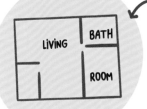

I'm good at misplacing things and bad at searching for misplaced items. That's why I always search room by room to avoid wasting time searching.

A friend bought me tracking tags because they understood my struggles with misplacing my things. I use one on my wireless earphones case, and it's working very well!

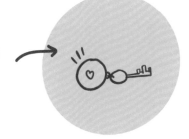

Being late

FOR MANY PEOPLE WiTH ADHD, BEiNG ON TiME iS NOT EASY

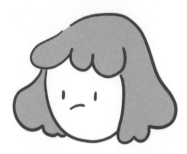

MY EXPERiENCE

I'm never on time. I'm either very early or very late. When I stress about being late for an appointment, I often leave my house way earlier than I should and overestimate the time I need to get there. When I'm super late, it's generally because I'm doing something interesting (like watching cute cats on TikTok), and I completely forget about the appointment until five minutes before I'm supposed to be there.

WHEN YOU'RE LATE BECAUSE OF YOUR LACK OF TIME AWARENESS

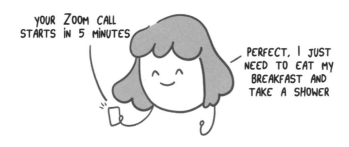

YOUR ZOOM CALL STARTS IN 5 MINUTES

PERFECT, I JUST NEED TO EAT MY BREAKFAST AND TAKE A SHOWER

WHEN YOU'RE EARLY BECAUSE YOU WERE AFRAID TO BE LATE...

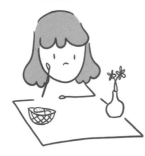

WHEN YOU'RE LATE BECAUSE YOU GOT DISTRACTED...

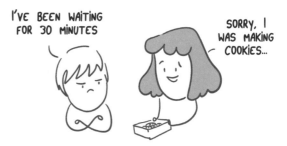

I'VE BEEN WAITING FOR 30 MINUTES

SORRY, I WAS MAKING COOKIES...

WHEN YOU'RE LATE BECAUSE YOU ANSWERED IMPULSIVELY...

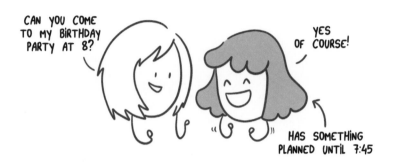

WHEN YOU'RE LATE BECAUSE YOU FORGOT YOUR APPOINTMENT...

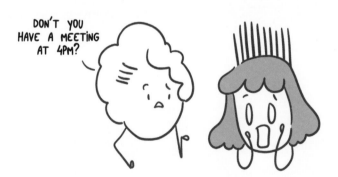

MY ADVICE

One or two hours before an important call or appointment, I try to limit distractions like social media or addictive TV shows. There are better times to start binge-watching!

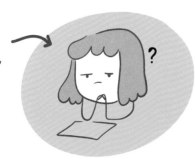

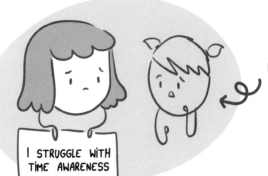

When I'm late, I apologize, but I also explain why I'm late. Not by saying that I got caught in an internet rabbit hole about the history of noodles, but by saying that I struggle with time awareness.

Driving

ADHD TRAITS LIKE DISTRACTIBILITY, INATTENTIVENESS, AND IMPULSIVITY CAN AFFECT DRIVING

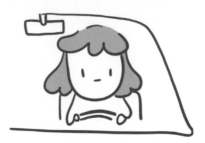

MY EXPERIENCE

For me, driving can be either extraordinarily overwhelming or a genuine pleasure. When I drive in the city and need to be careful of the signs, the bikes, and the pedestrians, I can quickly feel very anxious. Add to that somebody in the car with me or a GPS giving verbal instructions, and I'm completely lost. But at the same time, my impulsive brain thinks that driving fast (safely) on an empty motorway is one of the most satisfying things in the world.

...WE CAN HAVE TROUBLE PAYING ATTENTION TO TRAFFIC SIGNS

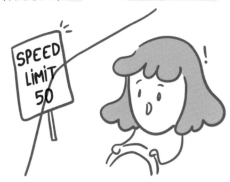

...WE CAN GET EASILY DISTRACTED, ESPECIALLY DURING LONG TRIPS...

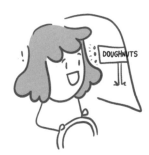

...OUR STRUGGLES TO REGULATE OUR EMOTIONS CAN LEAD TO ROAD RAGE...

...WE CAN HAVE TROUBLE FOCUSING
ON THE ROAD WHEN SOMEONE
IS TALKING TO US

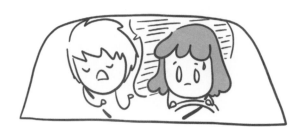

PEOPLE WITH ADHD TEND
TO BE AT GREATER RISK
FOR RECEIVING TRAFFIC
TICKETS

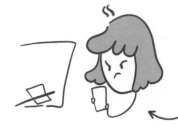

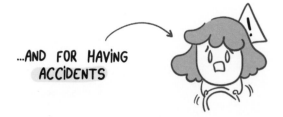

...AND FOR HAVING
ACCIDENTS

MY ADVICE

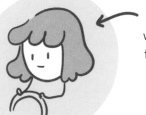

I try to reduce all distractions when I drive. I keep my phone, food, and anything interesting out of reach to help me focus on the road.

Since my ADHD diagnosis, I do not hesitate to tell my passengers that sometimes I need silence to be able to focus on the road.

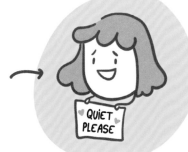

QUIET PLEASE

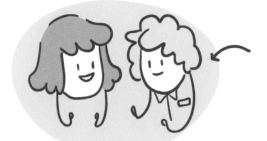

I consulted a therapist to deal with my driving anxiety. CBT exercises were very efficient in helping me feel more confident behind the wheel.

Texting

PEOPLE WITH ADHD CAN FACE
VARIOUS CHALLENGES WHILE
COMMUNICATING VIA TEXT MESSAGES...

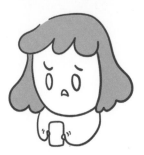

MY EXPERIENCE

Communication can be a big challenge for me, especially
texting. When I get a text message, I try to answer as soon
as possible, because if I don't, I know there's a good chance
I will just completely forget (yes, even though there is a
bright red notification icon on my phone)!

THEY CAN FORGET TO REPLY TO
MESSAGES AND ACCIDENTALLY GHOST
SOMEONE FOR WEEKS...

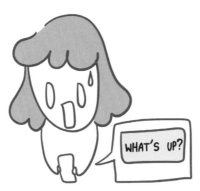

THEY CAN FEEL REJECTED
OVER A SIMPLE MESSAGE...

THEY CAN INTERRUPT WHAT THEY ARE
DOING TO RESPOND INSTANTLY TO AVOID
FORGETTING LATER...

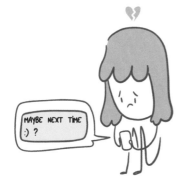

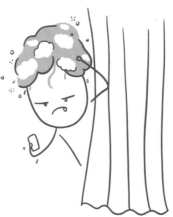

THEY CAN HYPERFOCUS ON A
CONVERSATION AND SEND THE
LONGEST MESSAGE...

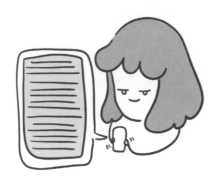

OR FOLLOW THEIR RACNIG
THOUGHTS AND SEND MANY
SMALL MESSAGES

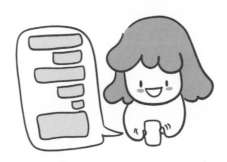

MY ADVICE

When I forget to respond to a text message,
I try to tell the truth. Since my diagnosis,
I have tried to explain my struggles.
I'm always surprised to see how understanding
people are when I simply tell them the truth.

If I know I can't answer a
text message right away,
I send a response like
"I received your text. I'll
respond as soon as I can,"
and I set a reminder for later.

SORRY, I FORGOT

To be sure I don't forget to
answer a message, I take a
few minutes each night to
go through all my messages.
If I don't feel like replying
instantly, I set a reminder for
the following day.

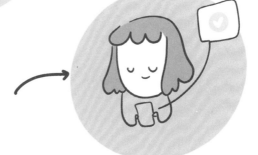

At work

ADHD SYMPTOMS IMPACT ALL
AREAS OF LIFE, INCLUDING WORK

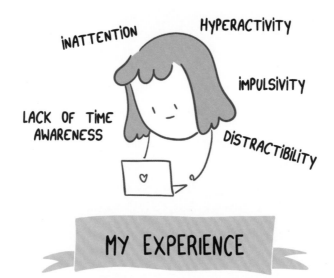

INATTENTION   HYPERACTIVITY

                              IMPULSIVITY

LACK OF TIME
AWARENESS   DISTRACTIBILITY

MY EXPERIENCE

I've had many jobs, and my ADHD symptoms were never
far away in every single one of them. As a hotel receptionist,
I dreaded guiding guests with verbal instructions, because
it was confusing, even when I was the one giving them.
As a freelance copywriter, I often had issues with my clients
because I made too many mistakes.

It can make us struggle to stay organized

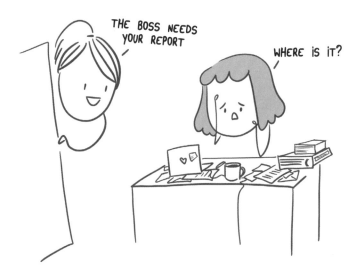

We can get bored quickly by repetitive tasks

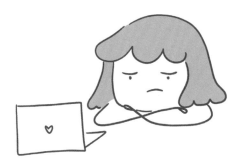

WE CAN GET CONFUSED BY VERBAL INSTRUCTIONS...

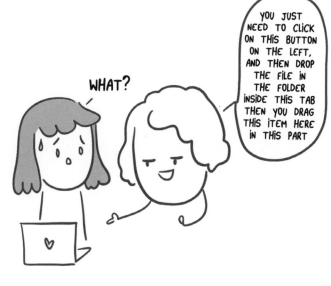

BUT WE CAN ALSO GET EXCITED BY NEW PROJECTS

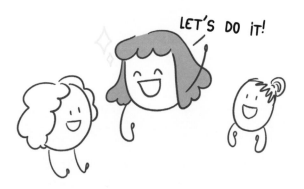

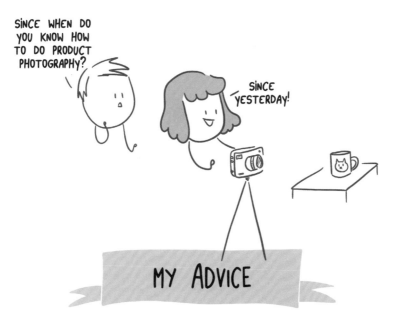

...AND LEARN FAST WHEN WE ARE INTERESTED!

SINCE WHEN DO YOU KNOW HOW TO DO PRODUCT PHOTOGRAPHY?

SINCE YESTERDAY!

MY ADVICE

Even before my diagnosis, I often asked for accommodations without realizing it was a way to compensate for my ADHD symptoms. For example, I often asked for a written document for essential instructions.

INSTRUCTIONS

BOSS

Becoming a freelance copywriter and then a content creator was one of my best decisions. Even though it's pretty stressful, it allows me to take advantage of my sudden bursts of motivation and inspiration while allowing myself time to do other things too.

Paperwork

MANY PEOPLE DiSLiKE DEALiNG
WiTH PAPERWORK. BUT FOR
PEOPLE WiTH ADHD, iT CAN
BE A REAL NiGHTMARE

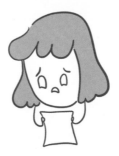

MY EXPERIENCE

I hate paperwork. I always have. I have unopened mail lying around, I'm waiting until the last minute to pay bills, and I'm lost every time I need to do admin stuff. All these things are utterly overwhelming, and I would be lying if I told you I've never cried with frustration trying to fill out an official form.

PAPERWORK WITH ADHD CAN
LOOK LIKE... HAVING A HUGE
PILE OF UNOPENED MAIL...

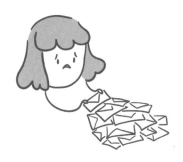

STRUGGLING WITH
ONLINE ADMIN TASKS...

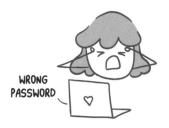

...FORGETTING TO PAY BILLS
(EVEN WHEN YOU HAVE
THE MONEY)...

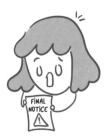

FALLING IN THE ADMIN AVOIDANCE SPIRAL...

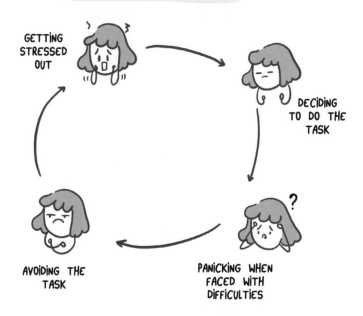

GETTING STRESSED OUT

DECIDING TO DO THE TASK

?

AVOIDING THE TASK

PANICKING WHEN FACED WITH DIFFICULTIES

IT'S EASY, YOU JUST NEED TO GO TO YOUR ACCOUNT ONLINE, DOWNLOAD THE FORM 67xP04, FILL IT, PRINT IT, AND BRING IT BACK ON THURSDAY BETWEEN 2 AND 4PM

GETTING OVERWHELMED BY "SIMPLE" ADMINISTRATIVE PROCESSES...

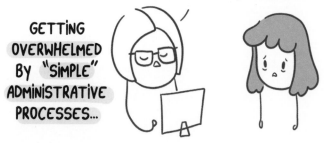

MY ADVICE

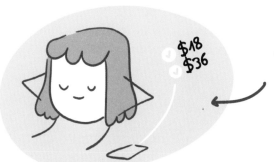

After paying another late fee, I decided to automate all my bills. It took some time, but now I know everything is paid for without my having to do anything.

I often ask for help when I feel like I can't do it alone. Having a friend helping me to understand how to pay my taxes or fill out a rental application always makes things easier.

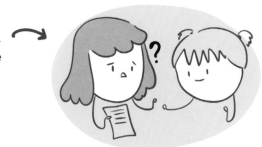

Deadlines

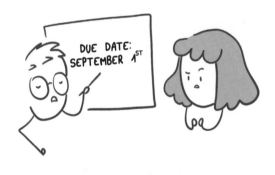

DEADLINES CAN BE QUITE CHALLENGING FOR ADHD BRAINS...

MY EXPERIENCE

I'm terrible with deadlines. When I have a deadline for something more than a few days ahead, I feel like I have all the time in the world to take care of the task. And, of course, I only realize I didn't do it right before it's due. This trait used to impact my professional life quite a lot.

AS WE TEND TO PERCEIVE
TIME DIFFERENTLY...

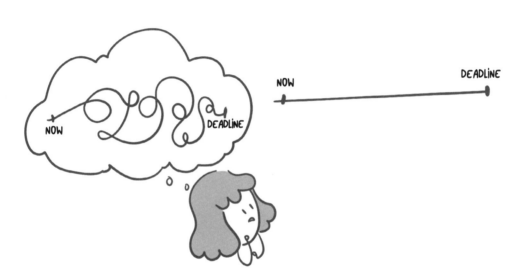

...WE CAN STRUGGLE TO PLAN AHEAD...

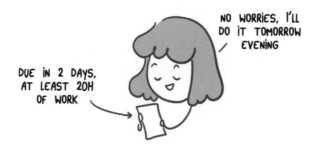

...AND WE CAN END UP RUSHING TO MEET DEADLINES AT THE LAST MINUTE...

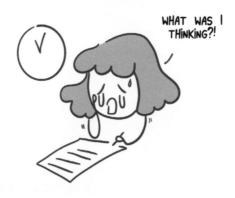

MY ADVICE

I always divide my work into small tasks that are more manageable. For example, if the first task is to write an email, but I'm having issues getting started, I sometimes set my goal as simply writing the subject line of the email. By making it easier to start tasks, I respect my deadlines better.

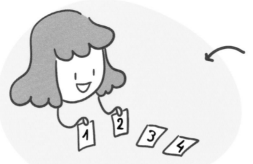

When I need to work towards a deadline, I create a visual tracking tool. It can be as simple as an arrow with steps on a piece of paper, or a table to fill on a whiteboard, but it helps me better understand my progress.

Working in batches always helps me start when I feel overwhelmed by the amount of work I have ahead. I'll tell you more about that in the last part of the book.

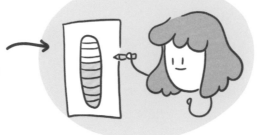

Food shopping

IT CAN BE HARD TO REMEMBER
WHAT YOU NEED TO BUY BECAUSE
YOU DIDN'T MAKE A LIST

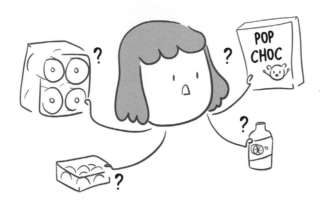

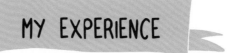

MY EXPERIENCE

Food shopping could be one of the daily tasks most impacted by my ADHD. Even with a list, I tend to get distracted and forget important items. I'm always buying fancy new stuff I don't need, and I can spend hours searching for something in the aisles, even though it's right under my nose.

...OR BECAUSE YOU FORGOT YOUR LIST

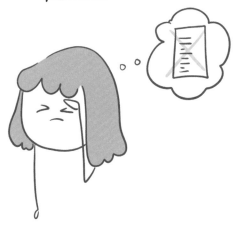

YOU CAN GET OVERWHELMED BECAUSE OF THE MANY SENSORY INPUTS...

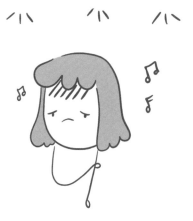

...HAVE TROUBLE MAKING A CHOICE BETWEEN TWO ITEMS...

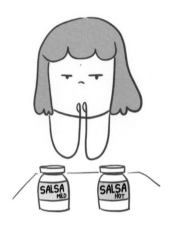

...OR IMPULSE BUY STUFF YOU DON'T NEED

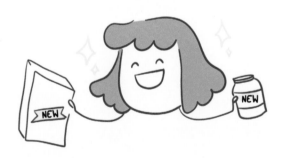

MY ADVICE

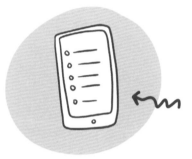

I'm way more efficient at food shopping since I replaced lists with checklists. I just made a checklist of all the items I often buy on my phone, and now I can use it every time I go shopping. I improve it each time, so it gets better and more detailed.

Grocery delivery is a lifesaver for me. I used to feel bad about not doing my shopping myself, but it helps me avoid forgetting things and be better organized at home.

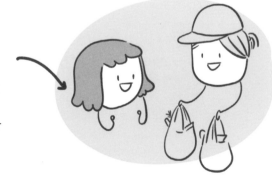

Hobbies

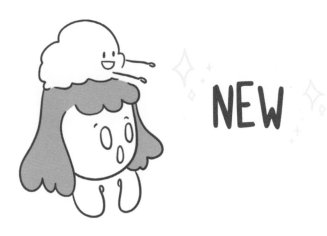

NEW

MY EXPERIENCE

I've always jumped from one hobby to another.
When I stumbled upon a YouTube video about roller skates,
I almost immediately ordered a pair online. I used them
every day for two weeks, and since then, they've never
seen daylight again. Growing up, I remember feeling quite
bad about being so "inconsistent" with my hobbies. Now I
tend to be more accepting of it as I know it's a widespread
trait among people with ADHD.

THAT'S WHY SO MANY PEOPLE
WITH **ADHD** REPORT ENGAGING
IN NEW HOBBIES VERY OFTEN

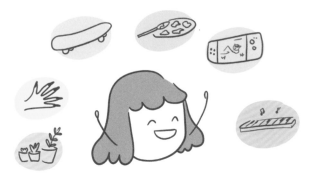

BUT BECAUSE OUR BRAINS ARE
PRONE TO BOREDOM...
WE ALSO OFTEN GET DISINTERESTED
IN THESE HOBBIES QUITE QUICKLY

UNFINISHED
PROJECT

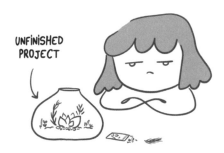

OTHER PEOPLE OFTEN MISUNDERSTAND THIS BEHAVIOR

WHY DID YOU QUIT PAINTING? YOU WERE SO TALENTED...

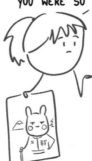 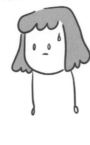

AND BEING MISUNDERSTOOD CAN BRING SHAME

WHY CAN'T I PERSEVERE IN ANYTHING?

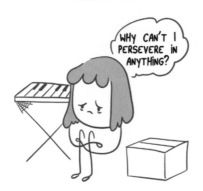

BUT, BECAUSE OF THIS TRAIT PEOPLE WITH ADHD OFTEN HAVE A LOT OF KNOWLEDGE ABOUT VARIOUS TOPICS

I'M A GLASSMAKER

THAT'S AWESOME! I TOOK A GLASSMAKING CLASS ONCE

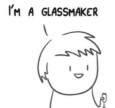

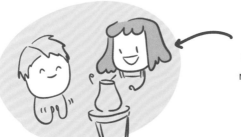

When I find a new hobby I like I try to find a club or classes to join. It helps me feel more accountable and not give up too quickly.

If I lose interest in a hobby I used to like, I sell or donate the supplies I bought. This way I don't feel bad about accumulating stuff I'm not using any more.

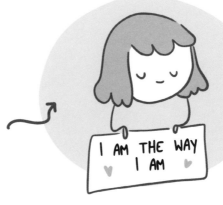

I AM THE WAY I AM

Exercising

WE OFTEN HEAR THAT
EXERCISE IS GOOD FOR
ADHD BRAINS

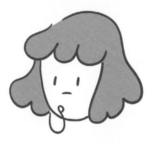

MY EXPERIENCE

For me, exercising can be enjoyable or feel like pure
torture. Practicing a sport I like, like badminton, is awesome
for having fun and unleashing some energy. But trying to
stick to a routine of something I find boring (like jogging)
is almost impossible.

...IT'S BECAUSE EXERCISE CAN HAVE A POSITIVE IMPACT ON SOME CHEMICALS IN OUR BRAIN...

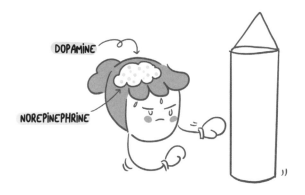

...SOME SPECIALISTS THINK THAT THESE CHEMICALS PLAY A PART IN WHAT MAKES ADHD BRAINS DIFFERENT

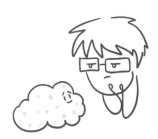

BUT EXERCISING CAN ALSO BE CHALLENGING FOR PEOPLE WITH ADHD

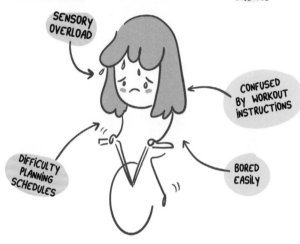

THE KEY IS TO DO SOMETHING YOU GENUINELY ENJOY

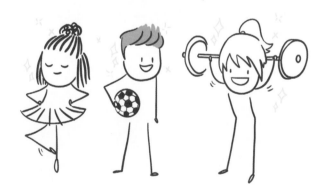

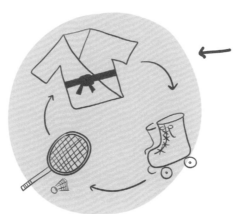

Now, I accept that I may need to switch activities often to enjoy myself while exercising. Of course, struggling with consistency might prevent me from getting a black belt in jiu-jitsu, but at least I can experiment with lots of different sports!

With physical activities, I don't force myself to do things I don't enjoy any more. I prefer to do something fun (like dancing to my favorite tune of the moment) and I end up forgetting it even counts as exercise.

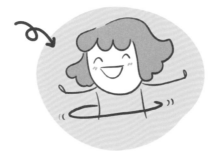

Tidying

MANY PEOPLE WiTH ADHD TEND TO BE A BiT MESSY

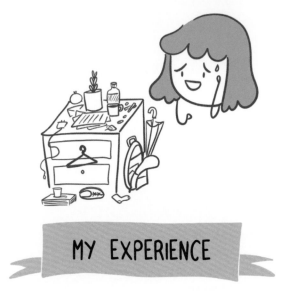

MY EXPERIENCE

Keeping my place tidy is quite a challenge. My home can become chaotic in the space of a day if I'm not careful. That's why I constantly try to pick up the stuff I've scattered all over the place. But as soon as I'm too tired or unmotivated to do it (this happens very often), I can quickly get overwhelmed by how many things are just lying around.

OUR PLACES CAN BECOME QUITE CHAOTIC AND WE CAN GET A BIT ASHAMED OF IT

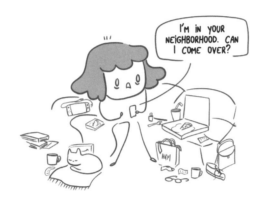

TIDYING CAN FEEL OVERWHELMING FOR ADHD BRAINS, AS WE CAN STRUGGLE WITH PRIORITIZING TASKS

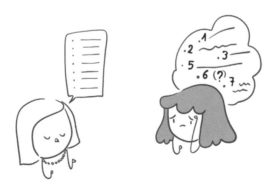

AND WE CAN EASILY GET
DISTRACTED BY THE PROCESS...

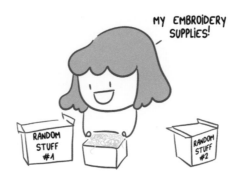

MY EMBROIDERY
SUPPLIES!

RANDOM
STUFF
#1

RANDOM
STUFF
#2

BUT LIVING IN A CHAOTIC
ENVIRONMENT CAN INCREASE
SOME ADHD STRUGGLES...

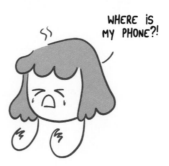

WHERE IS
MY PHONE?!

MY ADVICE

Being mindful of not purchasing too much stuff to avoid overcrowding my place is one of the best things I can do to keep my environment manageable.

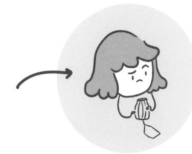

I try to take at least ten minutes every day to tidy my house.

I invite people over quite often. I know I'll get motivated to tidy and clean my place before my guests arrive!

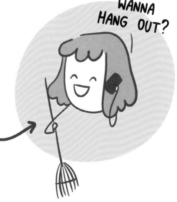

WANNA HANG OUT?

Dating

ADHD CAN IMPACT MANY SOCIAL ASPECTS OF OUR LIVES, INCLUDING DATING...

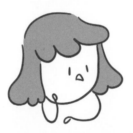

MY EXPERIENCE

Dating is nerve-racking for me. I know it's challenging for everyone, but for my ADHD brain, it's a whole other level. Some of my symptoms, like zoning out during conversations or interrupting people, are especially hard to manage when I'm stressed. I always feel either "too much" or bored during a date.

...EVEN iF WE LiKE SOMEONE,
OUR ADHD BRAIN CAN ZONE
OUT DURING A CONVERSATION...

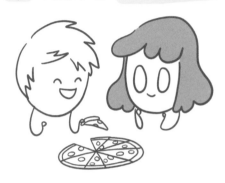

...WE CAN GET DiSTRACTED
BY MANY THINGS...

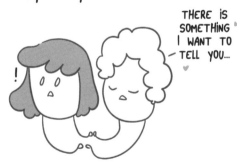

THERE iS
SOMETHING
I WANT TO
TELL YOU...

...WE CAN FALL FOR SOMEONE
VERY QUiCKLY...

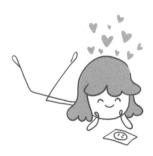

...AND STRUGGLE TO THINK
ABOUT ANYTHING ELSE

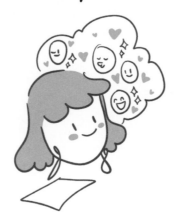

...OR GET BORED BY A CRUSH
AS QUICKLY AS WE FELL...

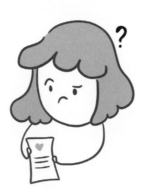

MY ADVICE

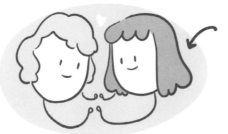

I find it very reassuring to see examples of people with ADHD who have great relationships. It proves that, even though ADHD can make things harder, it is possible.

Low self-esteem can exacerbate our dating struggles. Working on this, especially with therapy, before jumping headfirst into dates, helped me feel more confident.

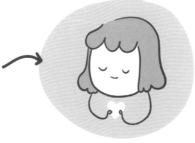

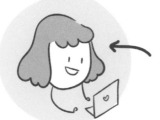

Talking to other people with ADHD online helped me feel less alone when struggling with unpleasant dating experiences.

Alcohol

PEOPLE WiTH **ADHD** CAN HAVE A
COMPLiCATED RELATiONSHiP WiTH ALCOHOL...

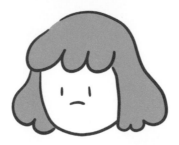

MY EXPERIENCE

Because I'm shy and I can be socially awkward, I got used to drinking when I met friends or new people. That was OK until life got a bit more stressful, and I noticed that I was developing a habit of drinking every evening to calm my nerves. Knowing that I have ADHD, I'm now cautious of my alcohol consumption, as I realize we have higher chances of developing an addiction.

AS THEY SOMETIMES STRUGGLE
WITH SOCIAL ANXIETY...

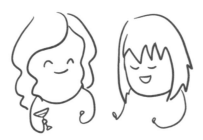

...PEOPLE WITH ADHD CAN TEND TO
DRINK MORE AT SOCIAL EVENTS

BUT MIXED WITH IMPULSIVITY, TOO
MUCH ALCOHOL CAN HAVE VERY
NEGATIVE CONSEQUENCES

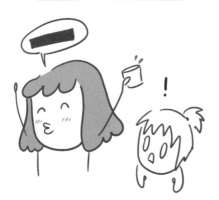

AS MANY PEOPLE WITH ADHD ALSO
STRUGGLE WITH LOW SELF-ESTEEM
AND DEPRESSION...

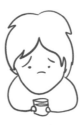

...ALCOHOL CAN FEEL LIKE AN
EFFECTIVE WAY TO NUMB
NEGATIVE EMOTIONS

BUT WE NEED TO BE AWARE THAT HAVING ADHD INCREASES RISK OF...

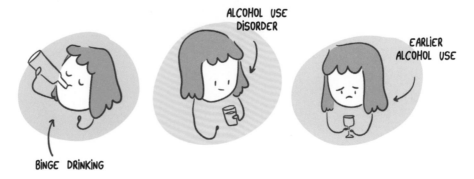

ALCOHOL USE DISORDER

EARLIER ALCOHOL USE

BINGE DRINKING

IF YOU ARE USING ALCOHOL TO REDUCE ANXIETY OR BECAUSE YOUR LIFE FEELS BORING:

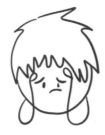

DON'T BE ASHAMED.
MANY PEOPLE ARE USING ALCOHOL AS SELF-MEDICATION OR AS A COPING MECHANISM

TRY TO UNDERSTAND WHY YOU DRINK

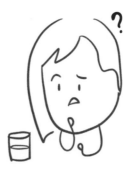

IF YOU CAN IDENTIFY YOUR PATTERNS, IT WILL BE EASIER TO FIND SOLUTIONS

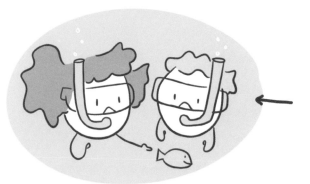

To avoid relying on alcohol to feel confident during social interactions, I try to do activities where alcohol is not an option (like playing sports or visiting a museum) with friends.

Therapy, and in particular CBT, helped me understand my triggers and develop healthier coping mechanisms.

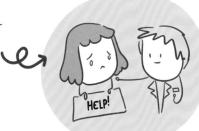

Making dinner

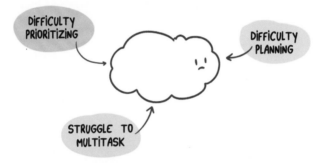

ADHD BRAINS OFTEN STRUGGLE WITH EXECUTIVE FUNCTIONS

DIFFICULTY PRIORITIZING

DIFFICULTY PLANNING

STRUGGLE TO MULTITASK

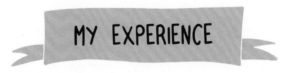

MY EXPERIENCE

I love cooking, but cooking with ADHD is quite a challenge.
I can't remember how many times I almost burned my
kitchen down because I forgot the oven was on. I'm not
bad at cooking meals from scratch, but following a specific
recipe, a cake, for example, feels almost impossible.

THIS CAN HAVE AN IMPACT ON MANY ASPECTS OF DAILY LIFE...

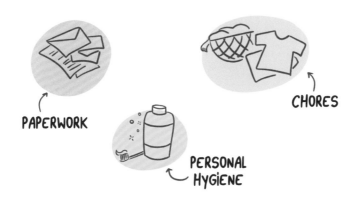

PAPERWORK

PERSONAL HYGIENE

CHORES

INCLUDING SOMETHING AS SIMPLE AS MAKING DINNER

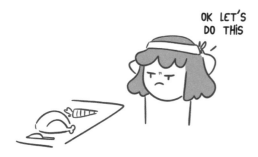

OK LET'S DO THIS

IT CAN MAKE IT DIFFICULT TO FOLLOW INSTRUCTIONS...

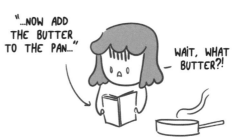

"...NOW ADD THE BUTTER TO THE PAN..."

WAIT, WHAT BUTTER?!

IT CAN MAKE IT DIFFICULT TO MANAGE SEVERAL TASKS SIMULTANEOUSLY

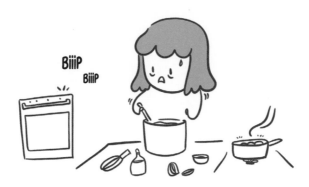

IT CAN MAKE IT DIFFICULT TO STAY FOCUSED ON THE RIGHT THING...

BUT WITH A BIT OF PRACTICE, SMART METHODS, AND HELP, ADHD BRAINS CAN BECOOME EXCELLENT COOKS!

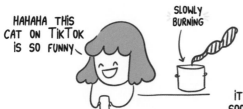

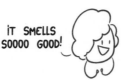

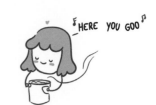

MY ADVICE

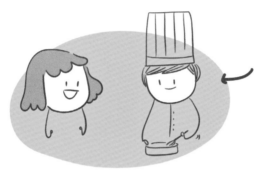

I took online cooking classes to learn basic cooking techniques, which helped me gain confidence. This means I can usually prepare delicious meals without struggling to follow a complicated recipe.

I try to take some time to cook when I feel like it and eat convenient things when I don't want to cook. By treating cooking like a hobby rather than a chore, I enjoy it more and more.

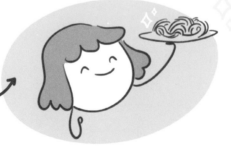

Binge eating

DID YOU KNOW THAT BINGE EATING DISORDER IS THE MOST COMMON EATING DISOORDER IN THE US?

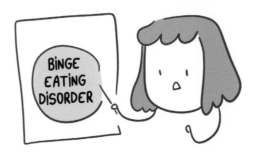

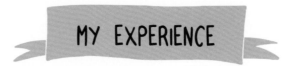

MY EXPERIENCE

Food is an easy way to reward myself when I have a hard day and I'm feeling low on dopamine. Whether it's comfort food from the cupboard (read: breakfast cereals for dinner) or a fast food delivery, food is always available to highlight the end of my day. But this habit of turning impulsively to food to feel better after a long day could lead to disordered eating.

ACCORDING TO THE NATIONAL EATING
DISORDERS ASSOCIATION,
BINGE EATING DISORDER IS
CHARACTERIZED BY:

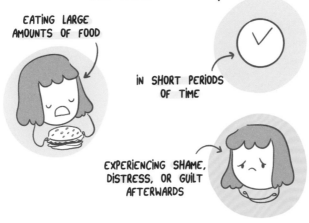

EATING LARGE
AMOUNTS OF FOOD

IN SHORT PERIODS
OF TIME

EXPERIENCING SHAME,
DISTRESS, OR GUILT
AFTERWARDS

PEOPLE WHO BINGE EAT OFTEN FEEL
AS IF THEY DON'T HAVE CONTROL
OVER HOW MUCH THEY EAT

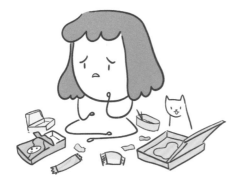

PEOPLE WITH ADHD ARE AT
INCREASED RISK OF EATING DISORDERS,
INCLUDING BULIMIA, ANOREXIA NERVOSA,
AND BINGE EATING

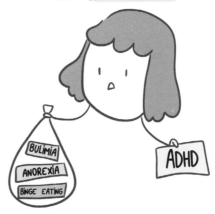

BULIMIA

ANOREXIA

BINGE EATING

ADHD

DUKE UNIVERSITY ESTIMATED THAT ABOUT 30 PERCENT OF ADULTS WITH BINGE EATING DISORDER ALSO HAVE ADHD

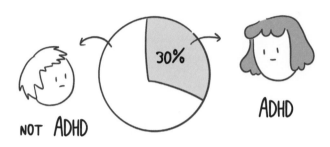

NOT ADHD

30%

ADHD

A STUDY FOUND THAT PEOPLE WITH ADHD COULD STRUGGLE WITH BINGE EATING BECAUSE OF A GREATER RESPONSE IN THE BRAIN'S REWARD SYSTEM

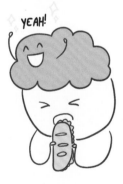

YEAH!

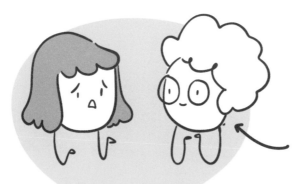

When I felt this habit was getting stronger and more challenging to avoid, I asked for help from my therapist. Together we were able to find better coping mechanisms (like enjoying a hobby) to deal with low dopamine at the end of the day.

My ADHD diagnosis helped me tremendously to better understand my relationship with food. Now I'm able to empathize with myself and feel less guilty.

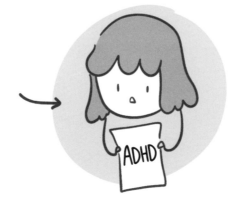

Video games

DID YOU KNOW THAT PEOPLE WITH **ADHD** CAN BE PARTICULARLY ATTRACTED TO VIDEO GAMES?

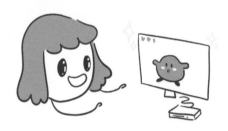

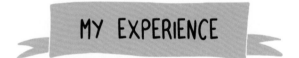

MY EXPERIENCE

I have always loved video games. When I was a teen, I could spend days building houses for my Sims. I was obsessed with that game. Now that I'm diagnosed, I understand that I was severely hyperfocusing on it! Today, I still get caught up in video games quite often. Even to the point where I forget to drink and take bathroom breaks!

IT CAN HELP US REGULATE OUR
PHYSICAL HYPERACTIVITY BY FIDGETING...

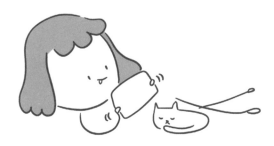

AND CALM OUR RACING MINDS
BY HYPERFOCUSING ON
SOMETHING STIMULATING

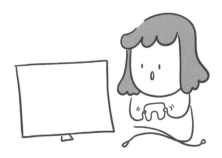

IN VIDEO GAMES WE ARE NOT
JUDGED FOR OUR MISTAKES...

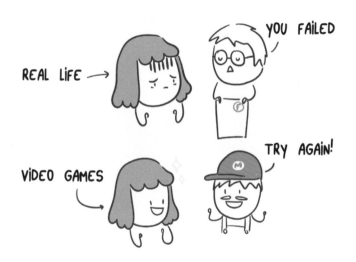

REAL LIFE → YOU FAILED

VIDEO GAMES → TRY AGAIN!

AND WE CAN MAKE FRIENDS THAT
SHARE OUR INTERESTS

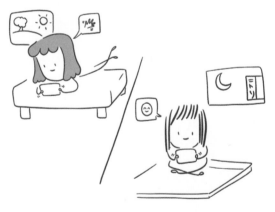

LAST IMPORTANT THING:
NO, VIDEO GAMES
DO NOT CAUSE ADHD

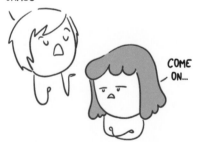

IT'S ALL THESE
VIDEO GAMES

COME ON...

MY ADVICE

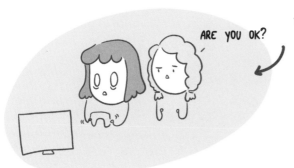

ARE YOU OK?

At some point in my life, when I was between jobs, I played video games too much. I guess it was the most exciting thing I could do, so I was pretty hooked. As people with ADHD, we should always be mindful of activities that can turn into addictions.

IT FEELS GREAT TO BE OUTSIDE

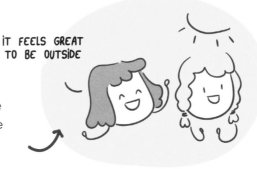

Today, I enjoy playing video games (even for long hours late at night), but I always make sure to do other things, too, like going outside for a walk and getting some fresh air.

Watching movies

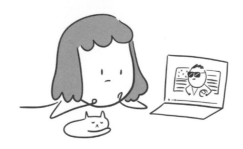

WATCHING A MOVIE, LIKE MANY OTHER
THINGS, REQUIRES MUCH ATTENTION

MY EXPERIENCE

Being a movie lover and having ADHD can have a
few pitfalls. If a movie or a TV show is not stimulating
enough, I quickly zone out, even if I'm enjoying it.
When I see an actor I think I know, I can't help but get
distracted and check their name, filmography, and Wikipedia
page. Then, of course, I need a snack. So, watching a movie
with my ADHD brain can take a while!

FOR AN **ADHD** BRAIN, IT CAN BE HARD TO STAY FOCUSED ON A MOVIE IF IT'S NOT STIMULATING ENOUGH

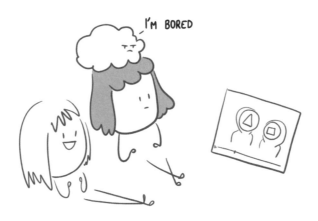

I'M BORED

IN THIS CASE, YOU MIGHT...

...MOVE A LOT AND KEEP CHANGING POSITIONS...

KEEP HITTING PAUSE TO LOOK UP INFORMATION ABOUT THE MOVIE

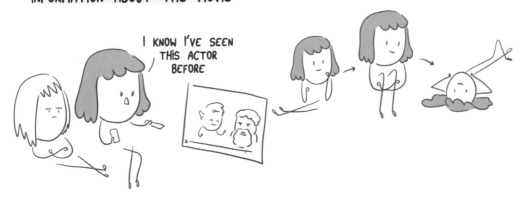

I KNOW I'VE SEEN THIS ACTOR BEFORE

...COMPENSATE FOR YOUR LACK OF STIMULATION BY EATING MINDLESSLY...

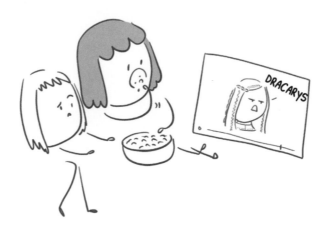

OR COMPLETELY ZONE OUT AND MISS HALF OF THE PLOT

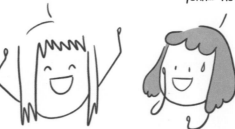

MY ADVICE

MY ADVICE

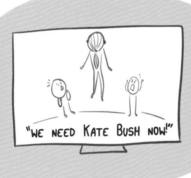

I often turn on subtitles on TV shows or movies to help me focus better on the dialogue. I zone out less frequently when I use this trick.

Sometimes, I need a few sittings to watch a movie or an episode of a TV show because I struggle to focus. When this happens, I don't force myself. Instead, I try to enjoy the rest of it at another moment.

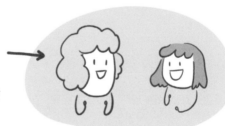

Intimacy

PEOPLE WITH **ADHD** CAN
FACE A VARIETY OF ISSUES
WHEN IT COMES TO INTIMACY

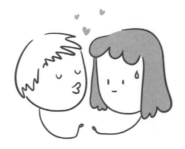

MY EXPERIENCE

When I first started to wonder if I had ADHD, I never
thought about how deeply it could impact all aspects of
my life, including my intimate relationships. Being easily
distracted during special moments is not fun, but it's easier
to accept when you (and your partner) know it's normal for
someone with ADHD.

OUR DISTRACTIBLE MINDS CAN
EASILY WANDER AWAY WHILE
WE ARE CUDDLING...

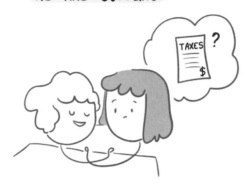

SENSORY SENSITIVITY
CAN GET IN THE WAY...

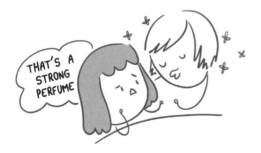

WE CAN ACT A BIT
TOO IMPULSIVELY...

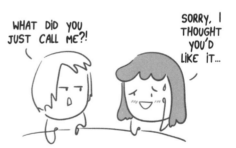

WE CAN GET BORED
DURING INTIMATE MOMENTS...

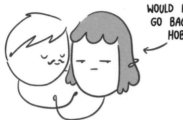

WOULD RATHER
GO BACK TO
HOBBY

OR EVEN BECOME
DISINTERESTED IN OUR PARTNER

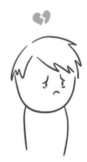

IT'S NOT YOU...

MANY PEOPLE WITH ADHD
ALSO REPORT DEALING WITH:

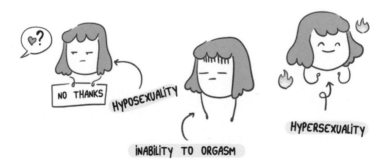

NO THANKS

HYPOSEXUALITY

INABILITY TO ORGASM

HYPERSEXUALITY

MY ADVICE

It might not sound very sexy, but I found that scheduling a special moment to share with my partner is one of the best ways to enjoy it without too many distractions.

Being sensitive to sensory inputs, I'm also meticulous about not having too many distracting factors, like strong fragrances or loud music, during intimate moments.

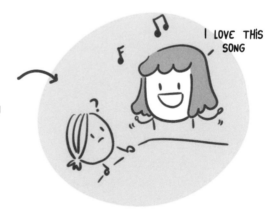

Bedtime

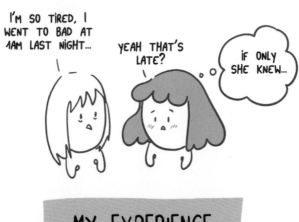

GOING TO BED AT A "REASONABLE" HOUR CAN BE A CHALLENGE FOR PEOPLE WITH ADHD...

I'M SO TIRED, I WENT TO BAD AT 1AM LAST NIGHT...

YEAH THAT'S LATE?

iF ONLY SHE KNEW...

MY EXPERIENCE

Bedtime was never easy for me when I was a child. I hated going to bed. I felt like I had so much energy! As an adult, it's still complicated. I often have ideas late at night, and I sometimes get caught up in creative activities that can keep me awake until dawn if I'm not careful. When I don't feel particularly inspired, I tend to scroll too much on social media and go to sleep quite late.

WE CAN EASILY GET CAUGHT IN FUN ACTIVITIES...

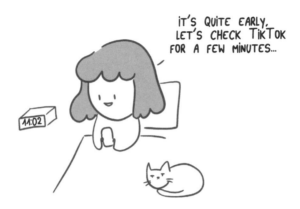

IT'S QUITE EARLY, LET'S CHECK TIKTOK FOR A FEW MINUTES...

11:02

...AND WE CAN HAVE TROUBLE KNOWING WHEN TO STOP...

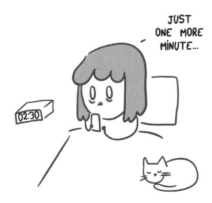

JUST ONE MORE MINUTE...

02:30

SOME PEOPLE WITH ADHD ALSO
FEEL MORE ENERGIZED AT NIGHT...

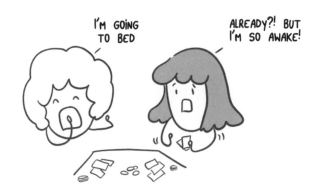

SOME PEOPLE WITH ADHD DREAD
BEDTIME BECAUSE OF THEIR
RACING THOUGHTS

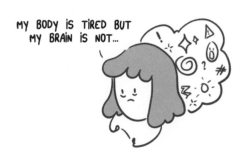

...AND OTHERS STRUGGLE WITH SLEEP
BECAUSE OF ADHD MEDICATION

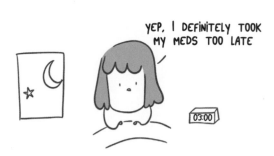

MY ADVICE

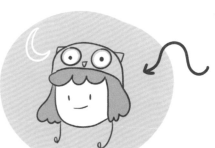

When I feel inspired or motivated to do something late at night, I try to go with the flow, especially if I don't have things to do early the next day. I enjoy being a night owl, and my diagnosis helped me to accept this part of my personality.

Staying away from technology (easier said than done, I know!) and engaging in screen-free activities like reading, journaling, drawing, or light physical activity help me feel more relaxed before bed.

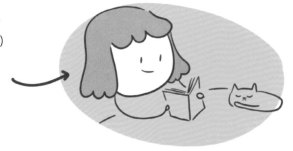

PART 3

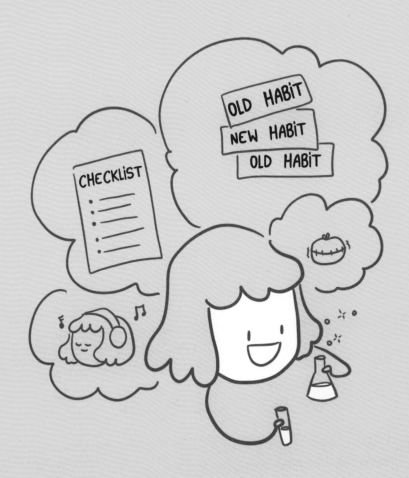

As we've just seen, life with ADHD can be very challenging. But I'm convinced that by using the right tools and strategies, we can eventually get things done and enjoy a more peaceful daily life. In this final part of the book, we will look at the key concepts and hacks that have helped me since my diagnosis. Not every single one of them will work for you, and that's OK. Try, learn, test things, and find the solutions that fit your life, not the other way around.

ADHD HACKS

Work smarter, not harder

"No pain, no gain" is not an ADHD-friendly mantra. People with ADHD should often aim for less effort and find smarter solutions.

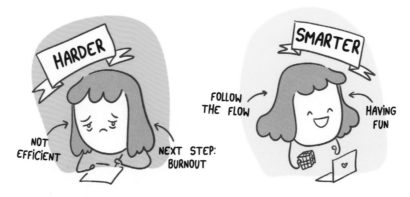

ADHD brains shouldn't have to "try harder." Making too much effort can sometimes signal that you are not using the right strategy for your brain. To achieve your goals and feel better, you could try instead to work smarter, not harder. Embracing this mindset will help you develop kindness towards yourself, and you'll also get better at finding creative solutions to your issues.

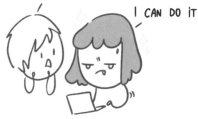

ONLY 20 MINUTES LEFT!

I CAN DO IT

If you know that you tend to work well under time pressure, it's OK to wait until the last moment to do something. As long as you make sure you've left enough time to complete the task, you will benefit from the pressure to get things done.

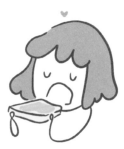

You don't have to work hard to eat well. Forget about complicated recipes and go back to the essentials. You'll see that great quality basic products, like in-season fruits or fresh dairy, don't need much effort to be delicious.

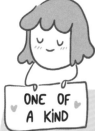

ONE OF A KIND

TIPS

There is rarely only one solution to a problem. Allow yourself to try a few things before finding the one that will work for you.

Take time to understand the issue and why you need to solve it before trying to find a solution.

Embrace your uniqueness. It's OK to solve things in a way that's different from how most people would.

"Hard work" is not always good work. You can be productive and creative without burning yourself out.

WORK HARD

HACK #2

Stack your habits

It should never be hard to create new habits! If you want to implement new rituals in your daily life, habit stacking is a great way to do it effortlessly.

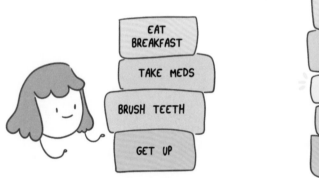
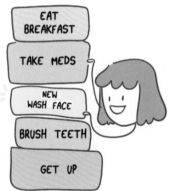

We all have habits in our lives. Even if your daily life looks pretty chaotic, there are still things you will be doing every day. These already existing habits are an excellent tool for creating new ones. Stacking new habits with your old ones will give them a better chance to stick. Try this first with simple things, and then, if it's working, see if you can add new habits every week or every month.

Clean your sink after brushing your teeth.

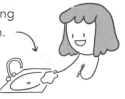

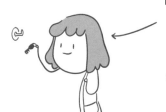

Put your keys where they belong as soon as you come home.

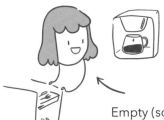

Empty (some of) your dishwasher while making coffee.

Take your medication when you turn off your alarm.

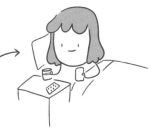

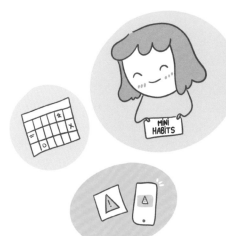

TIPS

Start small. It's OK to start with very simple new habits.

Use visual reminders (like sticky notes) and reminders on your phone for the first few days, so you don't forget your new habit.

Give your new habits time to stick before adding new ones.

HACK #3

Gamify your life

ADHD brains often crave rewards. As they tend to respond better to the carrot than to the stick, gamification is a great way to be more productive.

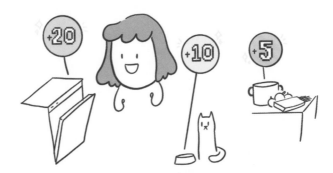

As we talked about earlier in the book, ADHD brains can be pretty motivated by video games! Have you ever noticed how gaming never feels like a chore? The time we can spend doing repetitive actions to gain points, coins, or any reward is quite impressive. So, why not use the same mechanisms in real life? There are many ways you can implement gamification in your daily life. You can give yourself points for chores, set rewards for tasks you really don't want to do, or even visualize the skills you want to develop, like a character from a game!

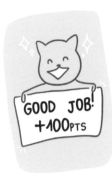

When you want to learn something, use apps that have an aspect of gamification. Gaining points, upping levels, and all the other little things can help you persevere with a task beyond the first impulse.

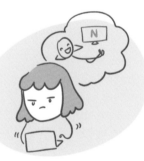

Set rewards for complex tasks. For example, allow yourself to binge-watch your favorite show when you did the dishes for three days straight.

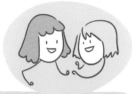

TIPS

It can be easy to skip the challenging tasks to go directly to the reward if you are doing it alone. Involve someone else in the process, so that you have accountability and will be less tempted to cheat!

Creating a gamification strategy for yourself can take time. It's OK if it doesn't work on the first attempt.

Set smart goals. To make gamification last, set realistic and meaningful goals that you want to accomplish with this strategy.

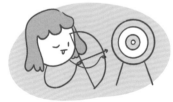

The Pomodoro Technique

Managing your energy and focus is not easy for someone with ADHD. That's where the Pomodoro Technique can be hugely helpful.

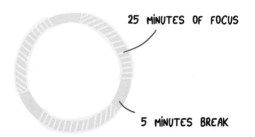

25 MINUTES OF FOCUS

5 MINUTES BREAK

People with ADHD often have an all-or-nothing approach. The ADHD brain can procrastinate until the last minute or hyperfocus to the point of forgetting to eat or go to the bathroom. The Pomodoro Technique is excellent for finding balance and getting things done. It works by defining a single task you want to work on (this can be a physical chore, an intellectual one, or even creative work). Then, work on this specific task for 25 minutes straight. After that, take a 5-minute break. Every four rounds, take a more extended 30-minute break.

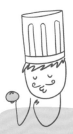

Next time you need to pay your bills or do admin work, try to use the Pomodoro Technique.

TIPS

We are all different. Feel free to test other Pomodoro durations to see if it's the right rhythm for you.

You can also use it for physical work such as cleaning and tidying your home.

Scan this QR code to watch my ADHD Pomodoro video on YouTube!

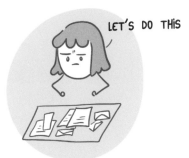

LET'S DO THIS

Don't neglect breaks! Like in sports, rest is as important as training. Breaks are part of the technique. Take them.

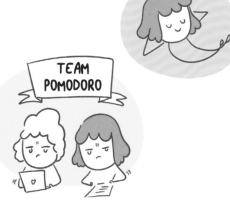

TEAM POMODORO

If you do it with someone else, the Pomodoro Technique is even more effective. But only if you are not distracting each other, of course!

HACK #5

Color-coding

ADHD brains often work better with visual cues. That's why color-coding some aspects of your life can improve your daily organization. And, bonus point, it looks awesome!

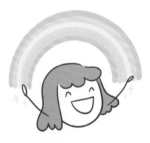

It almost seems too simple to be true, but trust me, color-coding can work tremendously well to help people with ADHD feel better organized. Universal and highly visual, colors can be an extremely powerful sorting system. If you close your eyes and think about an object you use daily, you will notice that you immediately know what color it is. If you use color-coding for daily organization, your brain will automatically know where to find it and where to put it back (maybe the most crucial part for ADHDers!).

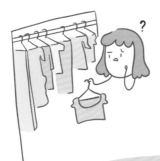

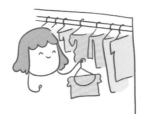

Organizing your clothes by color will give you a clearer view of your outfits. It's pleasing to the eye and will reduce the time you need to get dressed in the morning!

TIPS

Use colors to organize your papers: red for urgent, green for not urgent.

There is no limit to what you can organize by color: food in the fridge, laundry, makeup—anything!

Get creative, using paint, stickers, and washi tape to color-code your items.

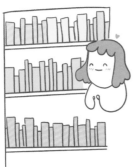

Sort your bookshelf by color. It will look beautiful, and you'll see that it will be much easier to keep it organized.

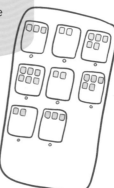

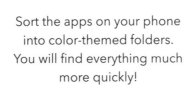

Sort the apps on your phone into color-themed folders. You will find everything much more quickly!

Work in batches

When you feel stuck in your to-do list, and it seems that you can't get anything done, batch working can help! Learning to work in batches, instead of trying to multitask, will boost your productivity, help you save time, and make you feel less overwhelmed.

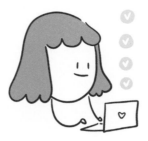

Instead of jumping from one task to another, staying focused on the same action will help you accomplish much more. As task initiation can sometimes be difficult for ADHD brains, working in batches eliminates this part of the equation, meaning you are less prone to procrastinate between tasks. It also reduces the risk of getting distracted and gives you a sense of momentum and achievement.

Batch cooking is an excellent way to eat homemade meals without the stress of cooking and cleaning your kitchen every day.

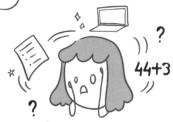

Need to clean the windows in your house? Try spending a set amount of time cleaning only the windows and nothing else.

Hate admin? Try setting aside one day per week where you do most of your admin tasks. This means you will have some peace of mind for the rest of the week.

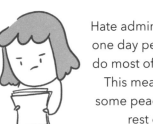

TIPS

If you have a recurring task in a week or month, set a day where you will focus only on this task.

Avoid scheduling meetings and calls during the time that you want to dedicate to batch work. The key is to work continuously without having a chance to get distracted.

HACK #7

Declutter often

Living with ADHD can get messy! If you want to feel less overwhelmed by your mess, I highly encourage you to declutter as often as possible.

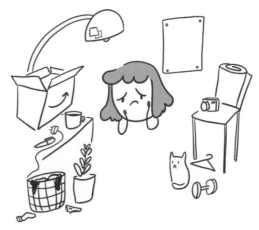

If you feel like your home is always in complete chaos, maybe one of the issues is that you have too much stuff. Between impulse buying and exploring many new hobbies each year, people with ADHD tend to accumulate a lot of things. The good news is, if you declutter often, you'll see that it will be much easier to keep your home (somewhat) organized.

Most of us have too many clothes. Don't be afraid to keep only the outfits you genuinely wear and get rid of the things that are always at the back of your wardrobe.

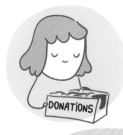

Declutter your electronics. Sell the high-tech gadgets before they lose their value and get rid of cables that belong to old or missing equipment.

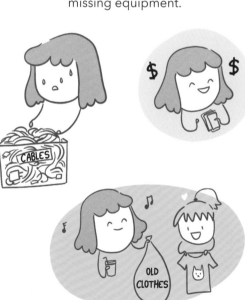

TIPS

Sell stuff that you bought impulsively. This can also help lower the ADHD tax.

Donate any clothing you haven't worn in the last year to charity.

Find a place for each thing in your home. If it doesn't have a place, maybe it should be donated or sold.

If you declutter often (every month, for example), you will see that it's not as overwhelming as it sounds.

Invite your friends over for a declutter party! It's a great way to find new owners for the items you don't need any more.

Find an accountability buddy

Committing to something, especially when it's a new habit, can be quite hard for people with ADHD. Having an accountability buddy is a very effective way of managing to do challenging things.

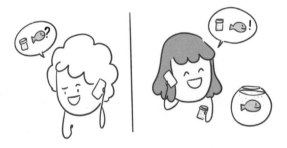

Because ADHD brains tend to handle motivation differently, it's helpful to find new ways to avoid quitting projects or dropping habits when things get challenging. Finding someone to help you stay accountable is hugely beneficial. You can commit to a daily text message to your best friend after you're done with your workout, send a picture of your clean dishes to your mother, or even join an accountability group online. The key is to use this strategy to do the things that are difficult for you until they are simply part of your daily life.

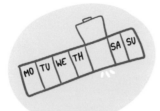

Struggle to remember to take your medication in the morning? Send a picture of your empty box to your accountability buddy every morning!

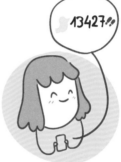

ACCOUNTABILITY BUDDY REQUEST

Hi _____

WOULD YOU LIKE TO BE MY ACCOUNTABILITY BUDDY FOR

_____ ?

LET'S DO A CHECK-IN EVERY:

DAY   WEEK   MONTH

ACCOUNTABILITY CAN HELP PEOPLE WITH ADHD ACHIEVE THEIR GOALS

Want to move more? Why not tweet your daily step count every day?

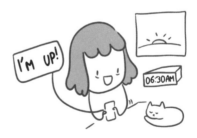

Trying to wake up earlier at the start of the day? Create a game with your best friend: the first one to text the other in the morning is the winner.

TIPS

If you struggle to build new habits and want to find your own accountability buddy, use my template!

Body doubling

Staying focused on a task can be challenging for people with ADHD. Body doubling can help you get things done by limiting procrastination and creating a feeling of accountability.

STUDIOUS ATMOSPHERE

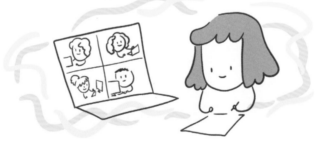

Body doubling simply means doing a task in the presence of someone else. Whether they are working on the same task or not, having someone else around often helps people with ADHD to focus. Body doubling can work in real life as well as online. You can use body doubling virtually by creating or joining a group of live meetings, or by watching videos on YouTube. I don't know why body doubling works so well, but it is worth trying!

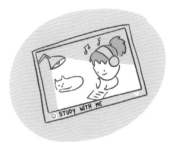

Watch "study with me" or "clean with me" videos to get motivated when you are alone.

Have a weekly virtual meeting with a friend to clean your homes while catching up.

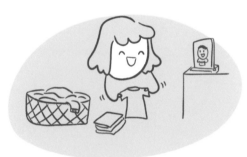

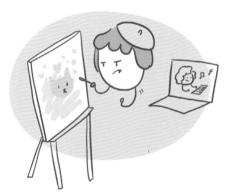

You can also use body doubling for creative tasks!

TIPS

Try to pair body doubling with the Pomodoro Technique.

If it works well for you, investing in a paid body doubling service to use this technique as much as possible could be interesting.

Label everything

Labelling is a great way to hack your brain. It will help you put your stuff where it belongs and avoid spending hours looking for something that you've misplaced.

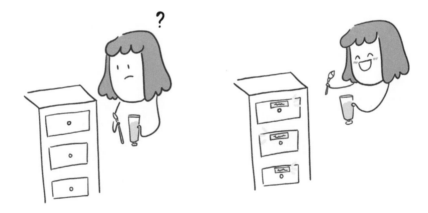

Putting labels on things can really improve your daily organization. Labels save your brain the effort of judging if somewhere is the right spot for the item you need to put away. If you do this for numerous things every day, you'll see that it will become much easier to keep your home tidy and prevent it from becoming complete chaos.

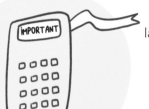

Medicine storage boxes with labels for each day help you avoid forgetting to take your meds, or stop you taking them twice.

TIPS

Invest in a good labelmaker. It will make labelling easier.

Practice makes perfect. If a specific label isn't helping you with your organization, try changing it for another category of item to see if that works better.

Do you like DIY projects? Try making your own labels to customize your decor!

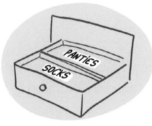

Is your wardrobe messy? Divide it into sections for different items and label each section.

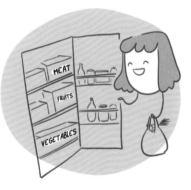

Put labels in your fridge! It's a challenging place to keep organized when you have ADHD. Using labels for food could be helpful.

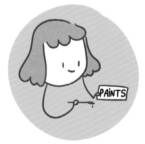

Brain dumping

ADHD brains can overflow with ideas and thoughts. Living with a mind that constantly feels full is not easy. That's why brain dumping is so effective in helping someone with ADHD to become less overwhelmed.

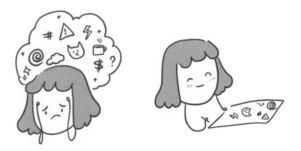

Brain dumping is quite simple. You just need a piece of paper and a pen, or your phone or computer. Then, write (or draw) anything that pops into your mind. This could be, for example, the bills you need to remember to pay, or the text message from your friend that you haven't replied to yet. Once it's done, you'll see that there's less stuff on the paper than you'd imagined. Then you can create a to-do list with these items, keep your brain dump as a reminder, or throw it away if you already feel better.

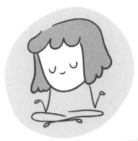

Try to get used to brain dumping as soon as you get overwhelmed or stressed out. You'll feel instantly more peaceful.

Get creative! Use colored pencils and pens to make it funnier and more engaging.

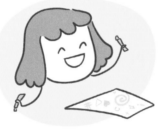

Brain dumping is not limited to work and chores. You can also brain dump personal stuff, like challenges in your relationships.

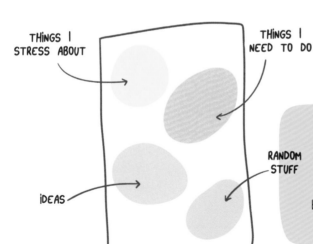

THINGS I STRESS ABOUT

THINGS I NEED TO DO

IDEAS

RANDOM STUFF

TIPS

If you struggle to brain dump on an empty page, use my template!

HACK #12

Identify friction

When you struggle to accomplish things or feel overwhelmed by the chaos in your life, take a break and analyze the situation. You will often find elements of friction that are making things complicated.

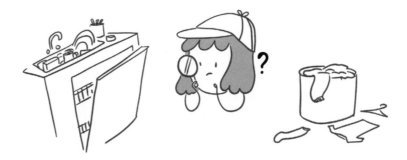

People with ADHD, especially those diagnosed as adults, are used to working against their brains. By masking and overcompensating, they get used to the idea that things should be challenging for them. In order to break this cycle and enjoy a much more peaceful life, you need to learn to identify the issues and processes that are incompatible with how your brain actually works. By eliminating this friction, you can do more and feel better.

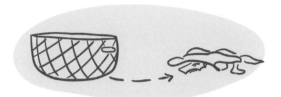

Are you tired of having dirty laundry in one spot in your room, instead of in the laundry basket at the opposite corner? The current solution is clearly not working for you. Try moving the laundry basket to where you naturally throw your dirty laundry.

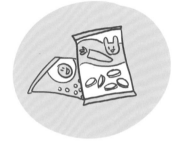

TIPS

When you see that a situation is not working well, analyze it to find the point of difficulty and remove it.

Don't be afraid to make your life easier. Choosing convenience is OK!

Try to avoid comparing your life to others' lives. Your goal is to make your life easier, not fit a Pinterest-worthy standard.

If the idea of washing and cutting vegetables is what prevents you from cooking homemade meals, buy pre-cut frozen vegetables. You don't have to make everything from scratch!

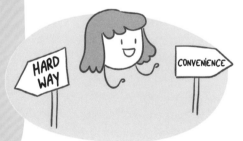

HACK #13

Use reminders

It may sound basic, but reminders can make a big difference for people with ADHD. Let's face it: it can be challenging to remember things when your brain is constantly distracted. That's why creating the habit of using reminders smartly can be powerful.

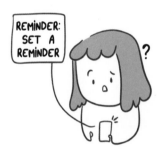

When you live with a very distractible brain, it's extremely easy to lose track of or forget things. Imagine you just remember that you need to respond to a friend's text. You pick up your phone, see an Instagram notification, and next thing you know, you've been scrolling on Instagram for an hour and you've unintentionally ghosted your friend. To avoid these situations, try to set reminders for important things you might forget.

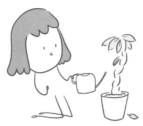

Your plants keep dying?
Set up a recurring reminder to
avoid forgetting to water them.

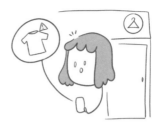

Some smartphones have location-
specific reminders. For example,
your phone could remind you to
pick up your clothes when you
walk by the dry cleaner.

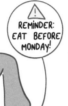

Set up a reminder when
you get back from grocery
shopping if some food
items are expiring soon.

TIPS

Reminders do not always work, and it's OK to
try something else. Maybe you could automate
this task (see how over the next few pages),
or stack it with another habit?

If you tend to not even notice reminders, try to
make them as loud and as visible as possible.
Use brightly colored paper when you create
physical reminders. You could also change the
sound of your alarm on your phone to be sure you
don't get used to it.

HACK #14

Use checklists

What's one thing that pilots, surgeons, and astronauts have in common? They use checklists! If they use this simple tool for doing such complex jobs, maybe we could learn from them. Creating checklists for important recurring tasks will help you gain time and avoid forgetting things.

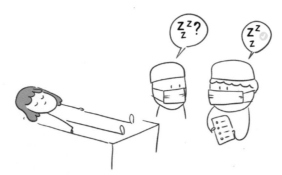

If you take a closer look, you will notice that many of our daily tasks are recurring ones. Taking the rubbish out, emptying the dishwasher, paying rent, brushing your teeth— all of these tasks are composed of actions that you've done many times before. This is why checklists can be extremely powerful tools for people with ADHD: you only have to create your checklist once and then you can use it as often as you want.

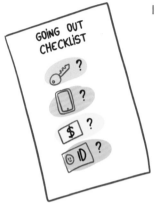

Instead of making a grocery list every time you go shopping, create a checklist with all the items you usually purchase.

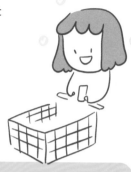

Create a checklist for leaving the house, to avoid forgetting important stuff. You can put it on your front door!

TIPS

Most smartphones have built-in tools to create simple checklists. Many apps are also available if you want something fancier or with more features.

Do you function better with physical tools? Create a checklist on paper and laminate it. You can reuse it as long as you want if you use a whiteboard marker.

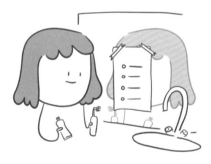

Do you struggle with hygiene? Create a checklist with your morning and night-time care routine!

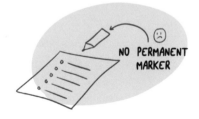

NO PERMANENT MARKER

HACK #15

Automate recurring tasks

Forgetfulness can be a daily struggle for people with ADHD. To fight it, some people spend every hour of the day concentrating on retaining information mentally, which can be exhausting and inefficient. Automating recurring tasks is a very effective way to improve your ADHD life.

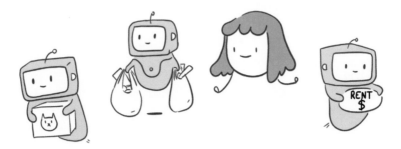

Do you often spend a whole day reminding yourself every 30 minutes that you need to do something, like ordering cat food? Well, automation could be a solution for you. When used correctly, automation allows you to limit the things you need to remember or manage, making your mind feel way lighter. Start by identifying the recurring tasks you struggle to remember, or those that take up a lot of mental space. Then see if and how you could automate them.

Automate all your bills and rent, and you will never pay late fees again!

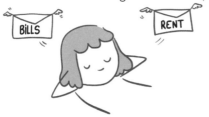

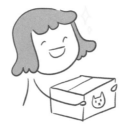

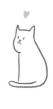

Use a subscription-based service to get some things automatically delivered, like cat food.

TIPS

Of course, automation is not a cure-all solution. You need to check in from time to time to see if the things you've automated work well for your needs.

There is no limit to what can be automated! Be creative and try things out. It's the only way to find what works for you.

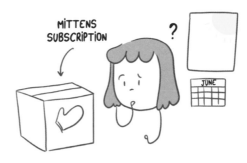

MITTENS SUBSCRIPTION

?

JUNE

Do you struggle to save money? Automate a regular transfer from your bank account to a savings account, or use an app that rounds up purchases to help you save money automatically.

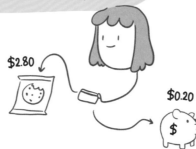

$2.80

$0.20

$

HACK #16

Use the power of music

Music is a powerful thing. It can make you sad, brighten your mood, or even help you focus. Using music to get things done might be one of the most simple yet efficient ADHD hacks around.

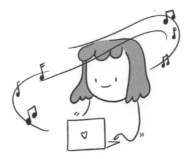

When you feel stuck in a task or unmotivated to do something, the most straightforward way to get things moving is to put on some music. Did you know that music has the power to increase your attention span? Listening to music you like increases dopamine levels in your brain, making you more attentive and motivated to finish something you've started. Music is also very useful for shifting your mood if you struggle with emotional dysregulation.

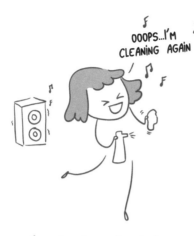

OOOPS...I'M CLEANING AGAIN

Are you struggling to meet a deadline for a project? Listen to a dramatic and uplifting movie soundtrack!

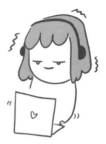

If you're struggling to keep your home tidy, put on your favorite song. Challenge yourself to clean as much as possible in the space of one song.

TIPS

Do you like to listen to the same song over and over again? This is very common among people with ADHD and is likely to be a form of auditory stimming.

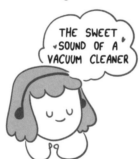

THE SWEET SOUND OF A VACUUM CLEANER

Stay mindful of your music consumption if you use headphones and if you like to listen loudly. It might help your brain, but you may hurt your ears!

If music is not working for you, try listening to low-frequency sounds such as white or brown noise. If you struggle to filter out background noise, these can help to you to regulate and refocus.

Scan this QR Code to listen to my focus playlist on YouTube!

Conclusion

Congrats, you made it to the end of this book!

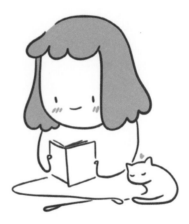

And it 's OK if you didn't read it in the "right" order! With this book, I wanted to create something you could use to find answers to your questions about ADHD, things like, "What's the ADHD tax?" A book that you could use to feel less alone when you experience something, like burning the dinner you were preparing for your date. And a book that you could use to find ideas for strategies to help you cope with some of your ADHD traits, like forgetting to pay your rent every month.

But, most of all, I wanted to create a book about ADHD made for people with ADHD. A book that didn't make you zone out (too much) because of long paragraphs; a book that felt accessible and fun. I hope I managed to do that. I hope this book will accompany you for many years, and that you can return to it when you feel confused, lost, or alone. I hope it feels like a safe place where you can be yourself. I wish for you to be at peace with your brain. You deserve it.

Acknowledgments

I am deeply grateful to all the individuals from around the world who have supported me on Instagram by liking, commenting, and sharing my posts. Your encouragement and kind messages have been incredibly heart-warming and have kept me motivated, especially when I was just starting my account and drawing on my phone with my finger (never let the lack of tools stop your creativity!). Your support has been invaluable in helping me continue drawing and posting, which is not easy for someone with ADHD.

D, without you, nothing would have been possible. I am truly blessed to have you in my life. Thank you for being you.

Baby D, your precious little kicks were my constant companion as I made this book. I feel incredibly blessed to be your mother.

Maman, thank you for always believing in me and giving me the strength to believe in myself. You nourished my creative brain with all your heart, and I'm sure you would have loved this book.

A heartfelt thank you to Morvan, Jemar, Janna, Christelle, and the entire TMAC Team for your unwavering support and encouragement. Your contributions have been invaluable in helping me manage our website and social media accounts.

I am deeply grateful to Hattie, my agent, for her kindness and patience. I also want to express my deepest appreciation to Sam, Evangeline, Faith, Emily, and Lucy, who have been the driving force behind this book coming to life.